The Nineteenth-Century Horse Doctor:

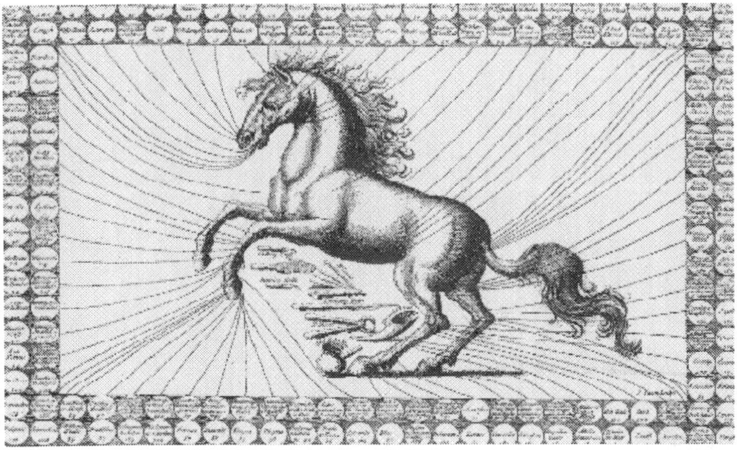

A Pennsylvania Dutchman's Practical Guide to Treating Horses

The Nineteenth-Century Horse Doctor:

A Pennsylvania Dutchman's Practical Guide to Treating Horses

NED D. HEINDEL & ROBERT D. RAPP

coffeetownpress
Seattle, WA

Published by Coffeetown Press
PO Box 70515
Seattle, WA 98127

For more information go to: www.coffeetownpress.com

Cover design by Sabrina Sun

The Nineteenth-Century Horse Doctor: A Pennsylvania Dutchman's Practical Guide to Treating Horses

ISBN: 978-1-60381-121-7 [Trade Paper]

Printed in the United States of America

The authors would like to thank Dr. Curtis Zillhardt and Samuel Stoltzfus for their valuable assistance in the preparation of this publication.

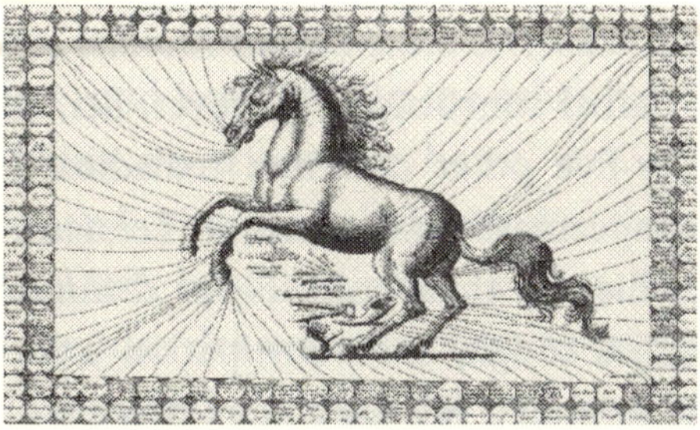

The first recorded house-by-house census in the colonies wasn't of people; it was of horses.[1] The horse was so essential that during the French and Indian War [1758], British colonial authorities ordered an ownership accounting in frontier areas so militia and armaments could be swiftly moved to combat areas on government appropriated horses. In towns, most shopkeepers and professionals also owned horses, and for both rural and urban folk, a horse was one of the highest value possessions. No immigrant German farmer could survive on his land without a horse. In one rural highly German township [Williams Township, Northampton County], the census takers found that each farmer owned at least one horse and twenty percent owned three or more. [2]

Little wonder, therefore, that books on how to keep one's horse healthy were among the most popular products of colonial printers. In the eighteenth century, as now, many ordinary Americans preferred using home medications drawn from a do-it-yourself book known as a "domestic physician" [in German, "haus arzt"] to the services of physicians. Germans in America probably got their first such book from the press of Benjamin Franklin, who in 1749 translated a popular English domestic physician written by John Tennent of Virginia, *Each Man his own Doctor: or, the Poor Planter's Physician.* Franklin's reprint, *Ein Jeder Sein*

Such was the medicine of Freitag's day. Whether treating his horse or his household, the farmer could use entirely herbal preparations, magic words, or a chemical formulation.

Freitag was so widely respected for his practical skills that in 1835, when local homeopaths organized a state-chartered medical school in Allentown—The North American Academy of Homeopathic Healing Arts—he was hired as one of the first four faculty members. At the first commencement in 1836, Freitag's three faculty colleagues bestowed upon him a medical degree for lifetime achievements. The diploma—printed in Latin, German, and English—is preserved in the archives of Hahnemann Hospital, Philadelphia. Shortly after receiving his doctorate, Freitag published a research paper in the *Correspondenzblatt der Homöopathischen Aerzte*, the official journal of the medical school. It was possibly his dissertation. [7]

The journal article was a case study of a single male patient suffering from a very difficult inflammation known as a fetid ozena. Ozena is a disease of the nose characterized by chronic swelling, wasting away of the bony ridges, and deterioration of the mucous membranes. Nasal crusting, discharge, and a very bad smell are other usual symptoms of ozena. Freitag reported that a precise formulation, dose, and frequency of administration of belladonna extract cured the condition. His book on home care of horses is similarly precise on the composition of the remedies, although sometimes lacking in the doses to be employed. Freitag was an unlikely author of a book devoted to horse care because, with a large medical and pharmacy practice, he would have had little time for large animal medicine. No historical information other than his book authorship ties him to veterinary practice. [5] Also curious is the fact that Freitag was an enthusiastic homeopath, committed to employing high dilutions mostly of botanical extracts—frequently in a spiritual or ritualistic context—and yet his *Deutsche Pferd Arzt* makes no mention of homeopathic principles and in fact teaches the use of various commercially available salts and plant materials in rather concentrated doses. [7] The tone that Freitag sets in his preface sounds like a plea for proper nutrition, good grooming, and tender care. He makes no claim for any especially valuable therapy but does, in fact, advance a rather strange claim for the origin of occasional blindness in foals. Freitag's *Der Deutsche Pferd Arzt* is clear and idiomatic, written for the German-speaking community of his day. Many of his terms for botanicals are of German origin. We have translated the Preface for Freitag's *Der Deutsche Pferd Arzt* and the entire text of Hassel's *Der Neuerfahrne Pferde Arzt.* By title, structure, and content it is probable that Hassel was building on Fretag's earlier text. However, as we have shown in tables that follow herein, the cures are markedly different.

Der Deutsche Pferd Arzt
Preface

For more than ten years I have received many requests both verbal and written from Germans to print a German language treatise on the common diseases of horses, including their diagnosis and treatment. Especially in the last few years, I have received requests begging me to describe in detail and make known the symptoms of the so-called "Gelb Wasser." I am attempting to satisfy their wishes with as much brevity and detail as my time allows.

Whoever uses this book correctly will not merely consult this and that page but rather read it from beginning to end. Moreover he should thoughtfully read the book through two or three times. If he hears that his neighbor or good friend has a sick horse, he should go to him, take his book, and determine the nature of the sickness by consulting this book.

Having done this and at the same time found immediately the proper medication and treatment of the horse, he will feel great satisfaction. If someone helps his neighbor in this manner, he will also please God.

Many people have asked me if I know of a material that can be used in the stall or applied to the horse to keep the horse healthy and prevent all sickness. The answer has always been and remains the same: groom your horse well. That is the best preventative medicine. One asks, what is the correct grooming of a horse? The answer is that grooming starts as soon as the foal is born. The first summer that the foal accompanies its mother, until St. Michael's Day or somewhat longer if the weather is mild. Then the foal must be weaned and placed in a stall with a low manger and a low feeding trough. He must be given the best hay and coarsely ground fodder. The reason for grinding the fodder is that by chewing the whole fodder, the foal distends the lower chin veins. This causes moisture and blood to be drawn into the eyes and hence results in blindness. There is no basis for the belief that the blindness of foals occurs because the fodder is not heated. No, the blindness is only due to the difficulty in chewing fodder that is not ground. It is even better if the foal is fed grain. Then one can be certain that the bones will not be thick and poorly formed; rather, the growth of the horse will be stronger and broader to suit him for hard work.

In beautiful weather allow the foal to run in the open air for one or two hours before putting him in the stall. Pay particular attention in wet and cold weather. This treatment, if adhered to, will produce a beautiful, healthy, useful horse. The horse must be at least three years old before being put to work. After the horse has done his day's work, bring him into a dry stall with an open front. An enclosed stall that is half buried underground and provided with shutters is very bad. This is why for several years now so many sicknesses prevail in Pennsylvania among horses. This treatment just described is the best preventative medicine against sickness.

The Editor, Bethlehem, Pennsylvania
December 1808

Freitag called himself 'the editor,' presumably because he admits that he was collecting sound veterinary advice from many sources. His publisher was Northampton County's most famous Pennsylvania German pressman, and likely his personal friend. Christian Jacob Huetter [Hütter] was a contemporary, seven years younger than Freitag. He had been born in 1771 in New Deitendorf in the German principalities but immigrated to Pennsylvania—where he was raised and later married—in Bethlehem, 1791. Huetter lived and worked in the Moravian community at the same time Freitag was its apothecary-physician. Huetter himself was probably not a practicing Moravian, for he belonged to the militia and rose to the battlefield rank of Lieutenant-General for the tri-county forces of Northampton, Lehigh, and Pike counties during the War of 1812. Until his 1849 death in Easton, where he had settled in 1808, his friends called him by his retirement rank of Colonel.

Huetter learned the printing craft and left Bethlehem to establish newspapers and publishing houses in Allentown, Lancaster, and Easton. While he mostly published German language newspapers, books, and broadsides, he also turned out a few English language products, and in 1810 he tried a bilingual newspaper, the *People's Instructor*, which ran advertisements and articles appearing in opposite columns in English and German. Neither the Germans nor the English speakers of Northampton County were ready for a totally non-political newspaper aimed to show them the language and problems of the co-habitating ethnic communities.

Our second manual—and the one translated completely herein—is devoted exclusively to animal medicine. *Der Neu-erfahrne Pferde Arzt,* by Carl Hassel, was published in 1843 in New Berlin, Union County, Pennsylvania. Hassel's book appeared thirty-four years after Freitag's thesis; nevertheless, it shows a strong resemblance in content and by the message of its title may have been intended as a later edition.

Here, little is known of the author, but considerable information is available about the printer. Joseph Miller opened a print shop about 1818 in New Berlin, one of the most thoroughly German communities in eastern Pennsylvania. New Berlin [originally Longstown] was surveyed in 1792 and in 1813 became the county seat of the newly organized Union County. Later politics relocated the court house to nearby Lewisburg. [8] Laid out on a 1774 land grant of 226 acres purchased by George Albright, a Dutchman from Lancaster County, this tiny town remained forty to fifty percent German from 1780 to 2000. The largely German protestant denomination, The Evangelical Church, was organized in New Berlin and maintained its official press in the town producing Bibles, hymnals, newspapers, and magazines such as *Der Christliche Botschafter*, *Der Antifreymaurer Advokat*, and *Des Freyen Volks.*[9]

While Miller published church materials, he used his press for certificates, posters, broadsides, and books, almost exclusively in German. For some he was both author and printer. In 1830 he published a very popular home medicine book entitled *Der Verborgene Arzt oder Nützliche Hausfreund* or *The Secret Physician or Useful Home Friend.* Devoid of occult cures, animal remedies, or the use of harsh chemicals, *Der Verborgene Arzt* takes the botanical Thomsonian system —then popular among New Englanders—and stresses how its mild herbal cures can help the Pennsylvania German farmer. Miller served as both author and publisher. In 1843, Miller reprinted the Hohman classic, *Der Lang Verborgene Freund*, as a verbatim plagiarism of the 1820 Reading edition with its mixture of occult and herbal cures for men and horses, and also the original Carl Hassel *Der Neu-erfahrne Pferde Arzt.*

The importance and widespread use of German language veterinary books in the first half of the nineteenth century is confirmed by the appearance in C.D. Lesher's edition of *The Citizen and Countryman's Experienced Farrier* [Chambersburg, 1841], a detailed German-English table of word equivalencies. Just as Hohman's pow-wow book for man and beast has seen more than 100 unauthorized reprintings and plagiarized re-editings, so *The Citizen and Countryman's Experienced Farrier*, an English bible exclusively for horse care, has seen dozens of reprintings and has been in circulation since its first printing in England in 1593 and edited reprinting in 1610. The author, Gervaise Markham, later cited as J. Markham, was a sixteenth century British poet whose books on country life included this famous one on horse care. American editions with additional authors and supplemental text began appearing almost a century after the author's death, in 1710, 1764, 1797, and 1841. The 1764 version, printed in Wilmington, Delaware, bore the strange credit line claiming authorship by J. Markham, G. Jeffries, and Discreet Indians. Apparently the first version to appear in Pennsylvania was *The Citizen and Countryman's Experienced Farrier*, supposedly authored by the long deceased J. Markham with the help of G. Jefferies and Experienced Indians. Somehow, between the 1764 version and this 1841 version, the unnamed Native American co-authors had ceased to be "discreet" and had become "experienced." This 1841 product came from the Chambersburg, Pennsylvania press of Thomas J. Wright and states on an inside foreword credit to one C. D. Lesher that this is the "republishing ... on account of the scarcity thereof" of the original edition, including a six-page table of "carefully added German names of the common plants and herbs made use of, which in any case is the principal part, so that you may not be at a loss to obtain the ingredients."

CITIZENS AND COUNTRYMAN'S

EXPERIENCED

FARRIER.

CONTAINING

A description of the Symptoms and Causes of the various diseases to which the Horse is liable,

AND

The most approved Remedies, employed in cureing of the same.

ALSO,

An experienced and approved method recommended in in the raising of Horses, as to their ordering, keeping &c., also, of Mares, Colts, and Stallions.

TO WHICH IS ADDED,

A list of the several Drugs and Herbs called for in this work, with their English and German names, and directions where they may be had.

BY J. MARKHAM, G. JEFFERIES, AND EXPERIENCED INDIANS.

CHAMBERSBURG:
PRINTED BY THOMAS J. WRIGHT.
1841.

This Lesher 1841 edition makes it clear that the farmer is more likely to find the necessary components to formulate the remedies by requesting them by their German names. The Table provides nearly 200 equivalencies including such examples as:

> adder's tongue [natter zuenglein]
> cumin seed [kummel], at the apothecaries [fennel seed may do]
> wild marjoram [wurst kraut]—ask for origanum at the apothecaries
> liver wort [leber kraut]—ask for lignum vitae guaiacum at the apothecaries
> juniper [wach holder] at the apothecaries
> turpentine [peintharz] commonly available
> verjuice [holz aepfel seider] the juice of wild crabapples
> nettles or dead-blind [taubo nesseln]

One remarkable aspect of Lesher's 200 therapeutic ingredients is the lack of agreement in the texts of that day on how to use these ingredients. Veterinary medicine was not a systematized professional discipline in the early nineteenth century. Commonly agreed therapies did not exist for the often-encountered diseases of horses. It is instructive to take four common diseases of horses and to compare author-recommended treatments for bots, glanders, yellow water, and lice.

Table of Comparative Remedies

Hassel	**Markham**	**Freitag**
	Yellow Water	
Valeria root	Aloes & English salts	Bleed the horse
Gentian root	Antimony	
Guaiacum	Flowers of sulfur	Mercury Acetate
Rhubarb	Copper sulfate	Jalap root
Jalap	Wood ashes	molasses
Red lead		
	Antimony	Potassium nitrate
	Flowers of sulfur	
	Camphor	Black snake root
	Juniper berries	
	Glanders	
Lard	Glauber's salt	Bleed the horse
Sap from rue	Saltpeter	Rye bran
Vinegar	Cream of tartar	Honey
	molasses	Chopped rye
Honey		Saltpeter
Oats		Chamomile
Exercise		Flax seed
		Wormwood
Arsenic trisulfide		
Fassiligens		

Table of Comparative Remedies (Continued)

Hassel	Markham	Freitag
	Bots	
Horse radish	Tincture of opium	
Milk	Turpentine	
Black pepper	Aloe	
Soot	Whiskey	
Sweet oil		
Turpentine		
Beeswax		
Mutton fat		
Sugar		
Urine		
Rum		
Pepper		
Gun powder		
	Lice	
Tobacco leaves	Parsley seed	
Mercury	Hellebore root	
Laurel oil		

This tabulation shows how different the concoctions are for these major diseases of horses. One quickly reaches the understanding that there was not one tried-and-true remedy which all the authors recognized for any one of these diseases.

However, one of the difficulties in comparing the recipes from author to author is that some texts simply list a series of apparently independent therapies while Freitag treats the disease with ascendingly powerful protocols. His description of glanders shows the concern for successful treatment of an animal ultimately tempered with the realization that a cure may not always be possible.

Glanders is a well known infectious disease in horses, mules, donkeys, goats, and occasionally cats and dogs. Twenty-first century veterinarians know it is caused by a highly contagious bacterium [Burkholderia mallei] often passaged in contaminated food or drinking water and manifested by nodular lesions in the lungs and ulceration of the mucous membranes in the upper respiratory tract. The animal coughs, displays a fever, and releases an infectious nasal discharge. Freitag includes these symptoms as an aid to his readers in diagnosing the condition: specifically he notes, Bei dieser Krankheit läuft ein verderbter Schleim aus der Nase ["In this disease one sees the production of foul-smelling slime from the nose."] He goes on to point out that the secretions can be white, yellow, green, black, gray or even bloody and that the nodules that are often evident under the ear or on the chin, head, neck, or root of the tongue must be drawn and drained or the animal will die. Professionals in animal care recognize that a general septicemia and death can occur within days of the appearance of the secretions and swellings. Freitag, of course, did not know of the existence of bacteria, and it isn't clear from his writings that he was aware that animal-to-animal infection occurred.

After determination that the horse has glanders, Freitag recommends that in a first step the animal be bled. Then one makes a mixture of one quart of rye bran, one quart of shredded rye, a gill of honey, and two ounces of saltpeter and feeds this to the animal morning and evening without interruption until the condition clears.

If, however, the problem persists, he next recommends a rebleeding and application of a medicinal formulation. A paste is prepared of finely ground solids—one-quarter pound of licorice and one-quarter pound of gum ammoniac [a basic plant sap, see item # 493, 14th edition Merck Index]—held together with two tablespoons of warm honey. The instructions say to form this into a well mixed large ball and then subdivide it into twelve small equal balls. Give one ball to the animal each morning after a night of fasting.

He goes on to specify that any accessible swelling must be drawn open, and for this another mixture of one handful each of chamomile, flax seed, and wormwood is required. With characteristic details reflecting his pharmacy training, Freitag requires this vegetable matter be heated with two quarts of water for one half hour and filtered while hot through a cloth. The nodules are washed with the warm fluid, and the warm plant matter that has been removed by filtration is pressed against the swelling. The desired outcome is that the swelling[s] have become larger and softer and have progressed to the stage of draining. Interestingly, although Freitag has no compunction about bleeding the animal, he does not recommend lancing the nodules.

If the condition persists—as evidenced by continuing nasal discharge—the owner must move rapidly to an inhalation steam bath. For this a ground-up mixture of one handful each of rosemary, marjoram, and pennyroyal is briefly heated in three quarts of water in a bucket, and the horse's nose is held over the vapors at least twice a day. To capture the aromas more efficiently, Freitag recommends that a large woolen blanket be used to cover the horse's head and the bucket. It is interesting that for some of these large volume aqueous preparations of botanicals—clearly intended for external use—Freitag deviates from his usual pattern of stating precise amounts. For these treatments of plant components in quarts or gallons of water, "handfuls" replace ounces and teaspoons as his measure of quantity.

If this inhalation therapy does not cure the condition and the nasal discharge continues, a spritzen solution is formulated for spraying up the animal's nose. For this concoction a handful of each of these botanicals—flax seed, elderberry blossom, and chamomile—is heated in three quarts of water, strained, mixed with two tablespoons of honey and one teaspoon of copper acetate and sprayed directly into the horse's nostril. While Freitag believed that this level of therapy would work, he also cautions that if the discharge continues as a black or foul-spelling fluid the owner must consider this as ein übles Zeichen [an evil sign] and progress to the last therapy.

The owner should retry the vapor inhaler and the nasal spritz while formulating one last potentially curative salve. This time one ounce each of liquid mercury and turpentine is thoroughly mixed with two ounces of hog lard and rubbed into all accessible swellings both morning and evening for fourteen days. If this procedure does not cure the condition, Freitag concludes that all subsequent help will be in vain. As he phrases it, Man schlache das Pferd lieber tod, or "Better that one strikes the animal dead" so that it no longer suffers and the owner does not invest needless money and effort on a cure.

Freitag's horse medicines and treatment protocols may have been described as more quantitative recipes than those found in other Pferde Arzt or Haus Arzt of the same period, but the ingredients he associated with a disease condition bore little congruency with those used by others. Such was the medicine of the day. Unsystematic concoctions of herbs and chemicals that varied widely from expert to expert had only one alternative—the magic words and occult manipulations widely accepted by the more superstitious farmer.

What does modern twenty-first century large animal veterinary medicine think of the concoctions in Hassel's and Freitag's books? Is there any merit to these antiquated treatments of rhubarb and molasses for colic, of black pepper, soot, and horseradish for bots, of garlic or onion for constipation, of mercury salts and tobacco for lice, of opium, turpentine, and whiskey for parasites, and of innumerable botanicals and minerals for founder, wound healing, poll evil, glanders, yellow water, and many other horse diseases? The *Merck Veterinary Manual* [Whitehouse Station, NJ, 2002] details the currently accepted therapeutics for more than fifty horse diseases, and almost none of them bear any similarities to those in Hassel and Freitag.

Whiskey and gun powder are nowhere to be found in Merck, but garlic and turpentine are. An oily ointment of garlic is used occasionally as an insect repellant. A few old-time farmers still apply turpentine and sometimes crude oil, carbon disulfide, or phenol as topical insecticides or presumptive treatments for insect bites in the horse. Practicing large animal veterinarians, however, recognize that such chemicals often induce exogenous hives that are more painful to the animal than the insect sting.

Opium itself appears to have no legitimate use; synthetic opioids are reserved primarily for analgesia. In addition, opioids are also employed as cough suppressants and for the treatment of diarrhea. Occasionally, opioids are used for animal sedation before surgery and as a supplement to anesthesia. Tincture of opium [commonly called paregoric] can be effective in staunching severe diarrhea, but it is more commonly given to dogs than horses.

The salt formulations so common in nineteenth century horse medicine—of lead, selenium, arsenic, phosphorus [phosphate], mercury, and other heavy metals—are today ranked as toxic to horses. In horses, lead salts or ingestion of lead shot usually produces a chronic syndrome characterized by weight loss, depression, weakness, colic, diarrhea, laryngeal or pharyngeal paralysis, and dysphagia, which frequently leads to aspiration pneumonia. Sodium borate is noted as a toxin, although frankly a rather mild and less dangerous one than many other inorganic chemicals.

Accidental ingestion by horses of vegetation such as acorns, potatoes, oleander, yew, thorn apples, oak leaves, tobacco, and many other botanicals causes toxicosis, often manifested as semi-formed and watery feces. There is no contemporary legitimate literature that justifies the use of nettles, crabapples, juniper berries, adder's tongue, cumin seeds, allspice, wild marjoram, and other plant materials often recommended in the Pennsylvania German manuals of the nineteenth century.

Bot therapies are still every bit as common in Merck in 2002 as they were in Freitag in 1809. Even in modern times there is still no satisfactory method to protect individual exposed horses from attack by the adult bot flies, but bot control programs, when applied on a regional basis to all horses, markedly reduce fly numbers and larval infections. The antiparasitic medicines, ivermectin and moxidectin, are the treatment of choice, for they attack the bot larvae in the horse's GI tract.

In founder or acute laminitis, the triggering condition must be corrected promptly. Today, founder is treated with analgesic anti-inflammatories [*e.g.*, phenylbutazone, meglumine, or aspirin]. Hosing or soaking the affected feet with pure cold water is also effective. Chronic laminitis with deformed hoofs is best treated by routine vigorous foot trimming and corrective shoeing by a skilled farrier.

The pharmacopeia of today's veterinarian is rich with the same kinds of synthetic pharmaceuticals used by physicians in human medicine. Sulfazine, sulfamonomethoxine, doxycycline, ceftrazidime, gentamicin, streptomycin, ephalosporin, fluoroquinolone, cloxacillin, oxacillin, amoxicillin-clavulanate, erythromycin, lincomycin, clindamycin, and chloramphenicol are but a few of the many standardized-dose pharmaceuticals used on horses. The precision of such rationally designed, carefully manufactured, and meticulously tested drugs delivered in pills or capsules has replaced the old German farmer's irrational empiricism, *e.g.*, a handful of pulverized horseradish root, a tablespoon of black pepper, and the pinch of chimney soot, boiled in a cup of sweet milk as a remedy for bots.

One big step in the transition from those empirical farmer- or farrier-generated, on-the-farm formulations to manufactured entities was the rise of the educated veterinarian, the professional horse doctor. The first veterinary schools were established in the late eighteenth and early nineteenth centuries in Europe, following waves of epidemics that killed an estimated 200 million cows between 1710 and 1750. Over thirty veterinary schools were founded in twelve European countries over a fifty-year period, including those at Lyon [1765], Vienna [1767], Turin [1769], Giessen [1777], Leipzig [1780], Bologna [1784], Budapest [1787], Munich [1790], London [1792], Madrid [1792], and

Edinburgh [1818]. In the U.S., Pennsylvania [1852], Massachusetts [1854], and New York [1857] had Colleges of Veterinary Medicine before the Civil War, and the great conflict stimulated others in Illinois, Missouri, Minnesota, and New Jersey over the next twenty years. The American Veterinary Medical Association was founded during the Civil War [1863] in New York by a French-trained veterinarian physician and its professional journal was published shortly thereafter.

Dr. Curtis Zillhardt, a retired Lancaster County veterinarian who practiced in Paradise, a rural farming community, remarked that such non-standard, haphazardly formulated recipes are no longer part of farm medicine. Zillhardt concluded that educated, professional veterinarians probably never used such therapeutics.

Dr. Lawrence Smith, a retired large animal veterinarian with the Bloomsburg Veterinary Hospital, recalled that as late as the third edition [1967] of the *Merck Veterinary Manual* there were still tables of suggested formulations reprinted in the book. Veterinarians at the time could whip up compounded therapeutics, even though commercially manufactured ones were widely available. Smith noted that by World War I, standardized and tested medications for a variety of horse diseases were available from a wide range of manufacturers, including Jensen-Salsbery [established 1913], Norden Laboratories [1918], Fort Dodge Animal Health [1912], Pitman Moore [founded before 1922], and Eaton Laboratories [ca 1885].

Even the government tried to help the movement toward rational large animal care and standardized therapeutics. The U.S. Department of Agriculture [USDA] in 1890 published *A Special Report on Diseases of the Horse*. Through reprintings and new editions—mainly 1896, 1903, 1916, and 1923—this

866-page volume remained widely available to practitioners for more than a century. Congress underwrote the original study and subsequent versions as a way to curry the farmer vote. USDA was commanded to print 100,000 copies, distributed according to a formula to all members of Congress, who would then provide them free upon request to farmers in their districts.

The 1916 edition is still available as a free e-copy [http://manybooks.net/titles/agricultureu2340323403-8.html]

In content covering cures and therapies, the 1916 edition of *Diseases of the Horse* stands historically at the cusp of the transition from farmer-empiricism to contemporary research-supported pharmaceuticals.

The complex botanical and toxic salts formulations of the eighteenth and nineteenth century farmer can still be found in this bible. Preparations containing tobacco, white oak bark, juniper, opium, colchicum, strychnine, asafetida, belladonna, cannabis, digitalis, arsenious acid, potassium chlorate, mercuric iodide, and potassium nitrate all sound suspiciously like the remedies found in Freitag and Hassel. And yet, the more modern veterinarian medications are invoked with equal frequency. Commercial drugs—synthesized, purified, and dispensed in standard dosage forms—are part of nearly every therapy. These include antipyrene, Lysol, chloral hydrate, quinine, camphor, salicylic acid, salvarsan, acetanilide, axytol, physiostigmine, theobromine, phenol, morphine, and others.

Bleeding and blistering were common in Freitag and Hassel, but are rarely found in *Diseases of the Horse* [1916], where most treatments are far less extreme, at least as starters. For example, a therapy to treat mange, a skin inflection caused by mites or microscopic acari, calls for scrubbing the skin with warm soapy water and a stiff brush and subsequently sponging on a dilute solution of tobacco boiled in water. The constipation of cramp colic is first to be treated by feeding natural laxatives, such as chopped apples and carrots, then by enemas of warm soapy water. Only if these techniques do not succeed are more heroic laxatives employed: ether and laudanum dissolved in a half-pint of linseed oil or powdered ginger root suspended in a half-pint of whiskey diluted by a pint of warm water. Cold showers and ice-water enemas are a first line treatment for fever. Feeding dry oats and dry hay is a stage-one treatment for diarrhea, but the ingestion of opium extract and bismuth subnitrate is available as a second line therapy. As a nod to the many German farmers likely to be using the *Diseases of the Horse*, the USDA authors used the German names for many of the diseases, *viz*, *Pferdestaupe* for equine influenza, *Brustseuche* for contagious pneumonia, and *Miltzbrand* for anthrax.

But old therapies die hard. As recently as forty years ago, some methods taught in the *Deutsche Pferd Arzt* were still in use among rural Pennsylvania German farmers. Smith, who started his veterinary practice in Quarryville, Lancaster County, recalled that he once encountered a large peeled onion inserted deeply up a horse's lower bowel. The Amish farmer was attempting to treat gas colic in his animal by irritating the intestine with the bulb. While the farmer looked on, Smith had to remove the onion with his arm inserted far up the horse before he could commence standard therapy [a gallon of light mineral oil laxative and an antispasmodic]. Smith also observed whiskey or ale used for equine viral influenza; turpentine and motor oil used for jagged wounds; lard used as a topical or uterine antibacterial; arsenic and strychnine in trace amounts for cattle who were "off their feed," and bull thistle tea for bovine pneumonia. Many of the cures were centuries old and, surprisingly, some of them appeared to work.

Smith remarked, "I never looked down my nose at farmers who used these primitive therapies or 'pooh-poohed' the recipes they used, even though they'd never have been my choice. In fact, in that case of the onion for colic, I cleaned off the bulb and reinserted it. The horse recovered, and I honestly don't know if it was the farmer's onion or my laxative. I've also observed some remarkable recoveries apparently affected by bull thistle tea. Some of those old remedies just might have worked."

For a snapshot of the development of twenty-first century horse doctoring, Freitag and Hassel represent the period of farmer empiricism. The USDA's 1890 *Report on the Diseases of the Horse* represents the first step toward modernity and toward current publications like the *Merck Veterinary Manual* [2002]. Today, equine veterinary practice has matured to embrace many specialized subjects. Highly focused textbooks now exist that deal with diseases in those specific organ systems in the horse: skin, skeletal, digestive, visual, reproductive, cardiovascular, and many others. Textbooks like *Large Animal Internal Medicine—National Veterinary Medical Series* [T. Ogilvie, J. R. Pringle, S. L. Ihle, and J. Lofstedt, Wiley-Blackwell Publishers], *Veterinary Pharmacology and Therapeutics* [J. E. Riviere and M. G. Papich, Wiley-Blackwell Publishers], and *Large Animal Internal Medicine* [B. P. Smith, Mosby Publishers] are just a few of the better known descendants of *Der Deutsche Pferd Arzt* and *Der Neu-erfahrne Pferde Arzt.* Freitag's and Hassel's treatises are worth remembering and reading as history but not as the standard of care for the equine medicine of today.

(1) Pennsylvania Archives, 5th Series, Vol. 1, *Horse and Wagon Census*
(2) Eighteenth Century Taxpayer Lists, Williams Township Supervisors, Easton, PA, 2000, p. 5
(3) Gerald Carson, *One for a Man: Two for a Horse,* Doubleday & Co., NY, 1961
(4) T. R. Brendle and C. W. Unger, *Folk Medicine of the Pennsylvania Germans: The Non-Occult Cures,* Proceedings of the Pennsylvania German Society, 45, 1935: pp 223-256
(5) G.B. Sowers, "The Private Notebook of Jacob Bucher, Jr.," *Der Reggeboge,* 2003, Vol. 37, pp. 3-9
(6) C. Waltman, *Eighteenth Century Bethlehem Medical Practices,* Oaks Printing, Bethlehem, PA. 1986: pp. 34-37
(7) G. Laubach and N. D. Heindel, "Homeopathic Medicine: Its Practitioners, Colleges, and Associations in Northampton County, PA.," in Vol. 9, *Bicentennial History of Northampton County,* Published by the Northampton County Bicentennial Commission, Easton, 1976, pp. 34-48
(8) F. A. Godcharles, "Chronicles of Central Pennsylvania," Lewis Historical Publishing Co, NY, 1944, Vol. III, pp. 379-380
(9) C. M. Snyder and J. W. Downie, *Union County: A Celebration of History,* Penn State University Press, University Park, PA., 2000, pp. 306-326
(10) This image is published with permission of the Historic Bethlehem [PA] Partnership

One of us [NDH] owns copies of the Hassel-Miller, Lesher-Wright, Freitag-Hutter, and Hohman texts cited above and the information given.

Der

Neu-erfahrne

Pferde-Arzt,

enthaltend 100

Curen und Recepte,

Originelle und ausgewählte,

Die als die bewährtesten im Lande bekannt sind.

Verfaßt von

Carl Zassel.

Neu-Berlin, Pa.

G. G. Miller, Drucker.

1843.

The Modern Horse-Doctor

Containing 100 Cures and Recipes

Original and Selected

They are known as the most proven in the land

Written by
Carl Hassel

New Berlin, Pa.

S.G. Miller, Printer

1843

sind; und siebenundfünfzig sind aus den bekannten besten Autoren gesammelt worden.

Die Namen der anempfohlenen Medizinen und Ingredienzen sind einfach und deutlich gemacht, und können daher von Allen verstanden werden.

Carl Hassel.

Franklin Caunty, Pa., März 28. 1843.

To a magnanimous public!

That there are many medicines for the various illnesses afflicting horses can not be denied; but in this as well as in other arts and sciences the possibility of making improvements must be acknowledged.

In this little book are contained a hundred recipes of which forty-three are original and if properly prepared and used are known to be effective.

There are also fifty-seven recipes collected from the best-known authors. The recommended medicines and ingredients are simple and easily prepared. The recipes can therefore be understood by everyone.

Carl Hassel
Franklin County, Pa. March 28, 1843

Nro. 1.

Gelbes Wasser.

Nimm 1 Unze Baldrianwurzel (Valerian root)
1 " Enzianwurzel (Gentian root)
1 " Gum (Guaiacum)
1 " Rhabarber (Rhubarb)
30 Gräne Jalappe (Jalap)
30 " Mennig (red lead)

Mische es und gib dem Pferde einen Theelöffel voll jeden Tag in den ersten drei Tagen der Woche. Wird es gegen das Ende der Woche nicht besser, so verfahre in der nächsten Woche auf die nämliche Weise. Ist das Blut am Ende der andern Woche noch nicht rein, so gib 3 Theelöffel voll anstatt einen.

Nro. 2.

Ein vortreffliches Pferdepulver zu bereiten.

Nimm 1 Pfund Spießglas
" 1 " Schwefelblüthe
" $\frac{1}{2}$ " Spice Berries
" $\frac{3}{4}$ " Bockshorn

Nr.1

Dirt malanders [a variety of eczema around the knee of a horse's foreleg]

Take 1 ounce Valerian Root
1 ounce Gentian Root
1 ounce Guaiacum
1 ounce Rhubarb
30 grains Jalap
30 grains Red lead

Mix the ingredients and give the horse a teaspoonful every day for the first three days of the week. If by the end of the week there is no improvement, repeat the next week in the same manner. If the blood is still not pure, give three teaspoonfuls instead of one.

Nr.2

To prepare an excellent horse-powder

Take 1 pound
1 pound Flowers of sulphur
1/2 Pound Spice Berries
3/4 Pound Hartshorn [Ammonium Carbonate, precursor to baking soda]

Mix the ingredients and give a teaspoonful every two days in the spring and fall as circumstances dictate.

— 6 —

Mische es und gib alle zwei Tage einen Theelöffel voll, im Früh= oder Spätjahr, wie es die Umstände erfodern.

Nro. 3.

Die Blut=Räude.

Nimm Salpeter, Schwefel, Weinsteinrahm, Salz, Harz; einen großen Theelöffel voll von jedem, thue alles in ein Peint Whiskey. Nachdem es aufgelöst ist, theile es in drei gleiche Theile ab, und gib einen Theil jede Stunde.

Nro. 4.

Wenn ein Pferd eine Schulter verrückt hat.

Nimm 2 Unzen Kampfer
" 2 " gemahlene Gewürznelken (Cloves)
" 2 " Terpentinöl

Thue alles in eine Quart Alcohol, lasse es 3 Tage stehen, dann wende es an und wasche damit zweimal des Tags.

Nr. 3

The bloody scabs

Place a large teaspoonful each of saltpeter, sulfur, Cream of Tartar and salt in a pint of whiskey. After it is dissolved, divide the mixture into three equal portions and give one portion every hour.

Nr. 4

If a horse has a shoulder out of order

Take 2 ounces camphor
2 ounces ground cloves
2 ounces turpentine

Place all the ingredients in a quart of alcohol and let it stand three days. Wash the shoulder with the preparation twice a day.

— 7 —

Nro. 5.

Für den Spath.

Nimm 1 Unze Brittisch Oel
" $3\frac{1}{2}$ " Vitriolöl
" 4 Tropfen Baumöl.

Thue das Baumöl (sweet oil) in eine Theetasse, tröpfele das Vitriolöl langsam darauf, alsdann gieße das brittische Oel dazu; thue die Mischung in eine starke Flasche und stelle sie auf heiße Asche, bis es kocht.

Anwendung. Reibe den beschädigten Theil mit einer Handvoll Stroh, bis er warm ist, alsdann nimm eine Feder und schmiere den Theil mit Obigem drei- oder viermal bei abnehmendem Monde.

Nro. 6.

Eine Salbe für Wunden und Geschwülste zu bereiten.

Nimm 8 Unzen Fischöl
" 8 " Terpentinöl
" 1 Eßlöffel voll Theer (tar).

Thue es zusammen und stelle es an die Sonne, bis es hell wird, so ist es fertig zum Gebrauch.

Nr. 5

For inflammation of the hock

Take 1 ounce British Oil [an essential oil]
3½ ounces vitriol [Blue, copper sulfate; White, zinc sulfate; Green, ferrous sulfate]
4 drops sweet oil

Place the sweet oil in a teacup and slowly drop in the vitriol. Then pour in the British oil. Place the mixture in a strong flask on hot ashes until the contents boil.

Use: Rub the affected part with a handful of straw until it is warm. Then take a feather and smear the part with the above three or four times by the waning moon.

Nr. 6

To prepare a salve for wounds and swellings [tumors]

Take 8 ounces fish oil
8 ounces turpentine
1 tablespoonful of tar

Put the ingredients together and place the mixture in the sun until it becomes clear. Then it is ready for use.

— 8 —

Nro. 7.

Wind-Kolik.

Nimm 1 Peint Molasses, ½ Unze Rhabarber, (Rhubarb). Mische und gib es auf einmal.

Nro. 8.

Ein Pulver zu machen für den Founder, das ist, wann ein Pferd überritten oder überfüttert ist 2c.

Nimm 1 Pfund Harz (rosin)
" 1 " Kupferwasser (copperas)
" 2 Unzen Bole Armenia.

Mache diese Artikel fein und mische sie; gib 3 Eßlöffel voll in warmem Wasser. Wenn es in 1 oder 2 Tagen nicht besser wird, so wiederhole es.

Nro. 9.

Eine Salbe zu machen für den Polibel, oder die Fistel.

Nimm 1 Unze Drachenblut
" 1 " Kampfer
" 2 " Schmalz (Hogslard).

Nr. 7

Wind colic

Take one pint of molasses and one-half ounce of rhubarb, mix the ingredients and give it at once.

Nr. 8

To make a powder for the founder [laminitis]; that is when a horse is ridden too hard or is over-fed

Take 1 pound rosin
1 pound copperas [a green hydrated ferrous sulfate, $FeSO_4.7H_2O$]
2 ounces Bole Armenia [a red variety of clay naturally containing ferric oxide and originally found in Armenia]

Grind the ingredients to a fine well-mixed powder. Give three tablespoonfuls in warm water. If it is not better in one to two days, then repeat.

Nr. 9

To make a salve for polibel [poll evil] or a fistula

Take 1 ounce Dragon Blood [red resin from middle and South American plants]
1 ounce camphor
2 ounces hogs lard

Mix and melt over a low flame. Use it twice a day.

— 9 —

Mische und schmelze es auf einem gelinden Feuer. Gebrauche es zweimal des Tags.

Nro. 10.

Eine Salbe zu machen für Ueberbeine, Klumpen und Verrenkungen.

Nimm 1 Unze Spanische Fliegen
" 2 " Blauen Vitriol [black
" 2 Theelöffel voll Lampenruß (Lamp-
" 1 Pfund Schmalz.

Mache die ersten 3 Artikel fein; schmelze das Schmalz, thue das Pulver hinein und rühre es bis es dick wird. Applicire die Salbe auf die beschädigten Theile; ist sie zu scharf, so mische Flachssamenöl und das Weiße von einem Ei, und reibe die Theile damit.

Bei Geschwülsten und Ueberbeinen (Wens), schneide die Haare weg und reibe die Salbe ein mit deiner Hand, bis der Theil warm wird, jede Stunde für 3 Stunden lang.

Nro. 11.

Für die Räude an den Füßen der Pferde.

Reibe die Füße wohl mit einem Welschkornkolben oder etwas anderem, bis der Grind all ab

Nr. 10

To make a salve for wens [boils], lumps [tumors] and dislocations

Take 1 ounce Spanish Fly
3 ounces Blue Vitriol [copper sulfate]
2 teaspoonfuls lamp black
1 pound hogs lard

Grind the first three ingredients to a fine powder; melt the lard and add the powder with stirring. Continue stirring until the mixture becomes viscous. Apply the salve to the affected part. If the salve is too sharp, mix linseed oil and the white of one egg and rub the part with it.

For swelling and wens, cut the hair away and rub on the salve with your hand until the part becomes warm. Do this every hour for three hours.

Nr. 11

For scabs on the feet of a horse

Rub the feet thoroughly with a corncob or something similar until the scab is completely removed. Then apply the best soft soap to the wounded part and bind it up. After three hours, wash the part with warm water. After the part is completely dry, rub it with hogs' lard.

— 10 —

ist, alsdann nimm von der besten Schmierseife, thue davon auf die wunden Theile und verbinde sie; nach drei Stunden nimm es ab, und wasche die Theile wohl mit warmen Spülwasser; wann die Theile ganz trocken sind, so reibe sie mit Schmalz.

Nro. 12.

Für die Hives.

Nimm ein Peint guten Essig und 3 Eier, mische es wohl. Diese Dose gib jeden Morgen, 3 Tage lang; alsdann nach 3 Tagen verfahre auf dieselbe Weise, bis du 9 Dosen gegeben hast.

Nro. 13.

Für die blinde Krankheit (blind distemper).

Nimm Salpeter, Alaun und Kupferwasser (copperas), gleiche Theile von jedem. Mache sie zu Pulver und mische sie. — Gib einen Theelöffel voll, für 3 Tage lang; alsdann nach 9 Tagen wiederhole es, bis eine Cur bewirkt ist.

Nro. 14.

Wann ein Pferd verstopft ist.

Nimm 1 Peint süße Milch und eine Hand voll Knoblauch (garlick); koche es zusammen; wann

Nr. 12

For hives

Mix thoroughly a pint of good vinegar and three eggs. Give this dose in the morning for three days. After three more days repeat the process. Continue in this way until nine doses have been given.

Nr. 13

For blind distemper

Take equal parts of saltpeter, alum and copperas and grind them together into a fine powder. Give a teaspoonful of this powder every day for three days. After nine days repeat until a cure is obtained.

Nr. 14

When a horse is constipated

Cook together one pint of sweet milk and a handful of garlic.

When it has cooled, give it to the horse.Repeat if necessary.

— 11 —

es kalt geworden ist, gib es dem Pferd. Wenns nothwendig ist, wiederhole es.

Nro. 15.

Für das Distemper.

Nimm ordinären Schnupftaback und geriebenen Meerrettig (horse radish), mische alles unter das Futter des kranken Pferdes. Es wird eine schnelle Cur bewirken.

Nro. 16.

Für den Engerling (bots).

Nimm eine Handvoll Meerrettig (garlick), koche es in einer Quart süße Milch, setze zu einen Eßlöffel voll schwarzen Pfeffer und einen Löffel voll Ruß (soot); nimm den Meerrettig heraus, und wann es kalt ist, gib es dem Pferd.

Nro. 17.

Eine andere Cur für den Engerling.

Gib dem Pferd ein halbes Peint Baumöl (sweet-oil).—Dies ist die beste Cur, die bekannt ist. Ein Tschill Terpentinöl ist auch sehr gut.

Nr. 15

For distemper

Take ordinary snuff tobacco and ground horseradish and mix with the fodder for the sick horse. This will affect a swift cure.

Nr. 16

For the bots [infestation of Botfly larvae]

Cook a handful of horseradish in a quart of sweet milk. Then add a tablespoonful black pepper and spoonful soot. Take the horseradish out and, when cool, give it to the horse.

Nr. 17

Another cure for bots

Give the horse one-half pint sweet oil. This is the best cure known. A gill of turpentine is also very good.

— 12 —

Nro. 18.

Für den braunen Wurm (im großen Darm).

Nimm einen Klumpen Pech von einer Fichte, so groß als ein Hühnerei; thue es in eine Quart Wasser und stelle es an einen warmen Ort, bis das Wasser davon stark geworden.— Gib dem Pferd ein Peint, ins Futter gemengt.

Nro. 19.

Für die Schwinden.

Nimm 1 Unze Kampfer
" 1 " Gewürznelken (cloves)
" 3 Köpfe rother Pfeffer
" 1 Handvoll Tischsalz.

Thue alles in eine Quart Whiskey, stelle es an die Sonne 2 Tage, alsdann schütte ein wenig in deine Hand und reibe damit den Theil recht gut. Dies ist eine unfehlbare Cur.

Nro. 20.

Cur für Wunden, geschehen durch Druck oder auf andere Weise.

Nimm eine Handvoll von der innern Rinde der weißen Eiche und halb so viel Camphrey

Nr. 18

For brown worms in the large intestine

Place a lump of pitch from a Spruce tree, about as large as a hen's egg, into a quart of water in a warm place. After the water has become dark, give the horse a pint mixed in his feed.

Nr. 19

For the swinden [Sweeney]

Take 1 ounce of camphor
1 ounce of cloves
3 heads of red pepper
1 handful of table salt

Place everything in a quart of whiskey and let it stand in the sun two days. Pour a little in your hand and rub the part vigorously. This is an absolute cure.

Nr. 20

Cure for wounds occurring due to pressure or in other ways

Take a handful of the inner bark of the white oak and half as much camphrey root [an herb]. Cook this in three quarts of water until one quart is evaporated. Then pour the liquid into an earthen container and add four ounces of alum. Let the mixture cool until lukewarm, stir well and wash the wound three times a day. After it is washed, smear the wound with mineral oil or Speiköl [oil from *Lavandula spica*].

— 13 —

Wurzeln; koche es in 8 Quart Wasser so lange, bis 1 Quart eingekocht ist; gieße alsdann das Flüssige in ein irdenes Gefäß, thue 4 Unzen Alaun dazu, laß es lauwarm werden und alsdann rühre es gut durcheinander. Wasche damit die Wunde dreimal des Tags. Mische Stein- und Speiköl zusammen, und schmiere damit die Wunde, nachdem sie gewaschen ist.

Nro. 21.

Für den Founder.

Nimm 2 Pfund weiße Wallnußrinde, thue sie in eine Gallone Wasser; koche es bis zur Hälfte ein, und wann es kalt geworden, gib dem Pferd eine Quart; nach 10 Stunden (wenns nöthig ist) gib die andere Quart.

Nro. 22.

Für den Engerling(bots).

Nimm fünf Nux vomeca (french buttons) feile sie zu Pulver, thue es in eine Quartflasche und fülle sie mit warmen Wasser an.—Gib dem Pferd davon ein.

Nr.21

For the founder

Take two pounds. of white walnut shells and place them into a gallon of water. Cook it until the volume has decreased by one half. When it is cold give the horse one quart. After ten hours, if it is necessary, give the other quart.

Nr. 22

For the bots

Take five Nux vomica nuts [French buttons] and file them to a powder in a quart vessel. Fill the container with warm water and give to the horse.

— 14 —

Nro. 23.

Um die Würmer zu verhüten.

Gib deinem Pferde eine große Handvoll Rainfarn (tansy), grün oder getrocknet, drei- oder viermal des Jahrs.—Es ist auch sehr gut für die Windkolik.

Nro. 24.

Für die Hives.

Nimm einen Mink, thue ihn in ein irdenes Gefäß und stelle es bedeckt in einen Backofen, der heiß genug ist um Brod zu backen; wiederhole es, bis der Mink zu Kohle gebrannt ist. Pulverisire ihn alsdann und gib dem Pferde einen Theelöffel voll davon Morgens und Abends.

Nro. 25.

Für den Husten.

Nimm 5 Hühnereier, weiche sie in starkem Essig ein, bis die Schalen weich sind; ziehe die Zunge des Pferdes auf eine Seite, wirf die Eier in seinen Hals und mache, daß er sie hinunterschluckt. Wiederhole es, wenn nöthig.

Nr. 23

In order to prevent worms

Give to your horse a large handful of green or dried Tansy three or four times per year. It is also very good for wind cholic.

Nr. 24

For hives

Place a mink in a covered earthen container and place it in a bake oven that is hot enough to bake bread. Repeat until the mink is burned to charcoal. Then pulverize it and give a teaspoonful morning and evening.

Nr. 25

For coughs

Soak five hen's eggs in strong vinegar until the shells are soft. Pull the tongue of the horse to one side and put the eggs into his throat and make him swallow them. Repeat this as necessary.

— 15 —

Nro. 26.

Ein anderes für den Husten.

Nimm eine Handvoll Lungenkraut
" 2 Unzen Haselwurzel (hazelroot).
" 2 Quart Gerste.

Thue alles in 3 Gallone Wasser und koche es ein bis auf zwei.—Gib dem Pferde täglich eine Quart und laß es alsdann zur Ader.

Nro. 27.

Für die Kolik.

Nimm einen Eßlöffel voll Senf- oder Rübensamen, und mache denselben fein. Gib es in einem halben Peint Rum oder Tschin.

Nro. 28.

Für die Windkolik.

Nimm eine große Handvoll von der Rinde der Aspe, thue es in einen Hafen, schütte eine halbe Gallon Wasser darauf und koche es ein bis zur Hälfte; schütte alsdann das Flüssige in ein anderes Gefäß. Wann es lauwarm ist, tränke das Pferd damit, und reite oder führe es eine kurze Zeit umher.

Nr. 26

Another for coughs

Take a handful of Lungenkraut [*Pulmonaria officianalis*]
2 ounces of Hazel root
2 quarts of Barley

Put everything in three gallons of water and cook until the volume is reduced to two gallons. Give the horse one-quart daily and then bleed him.

Nr. 27

For colic

Take a tablespoonful of mustard or rape seed and pulverize it. Give this in a half pint of rum or Ischin [Ischin is a variety of green fig that ripens in July and August, and this remedy probably refers to an alcoholic drink made from this fruit].

Nr. 28

For the wind colic

Take a large handful of the bark of the Aspen and place it in a pot. Pour over this a half-gallon of water and cook until the volume is reduced to half. Then pour the liquid into another container to cool. When it is lukewarm, give it to the horse to drink and ride or lead the horse around for a short time.

— 16 —

Nro. 26.

Wann ein Pferd überhitzt ist.

Nimm ½ Peint Flachssamenöl
" ½ " Schmalz.

Mische es;—gib es dem Pferd und wasche es mit frischem Wasser.

Nro. 30.

Für eine Geschwulst.

Nimm Silberglätte und guten Essig, von jedem gleich viel und mische es; nachdem es eine Stunde gestanden, gieße Baumöl (sweet oil) darauf, bis es dünn wird.—Schmiere damit den geschwollenen Theil.

Nro. 31.

Eine vortreffliche Salbe zu machen, die irgend eine Wunde heilt, sie mag verursacht seyn durch den Sattel, das Kummet oder irgend sonst etwas.

Nimm 2 Unzen vom Fett (grease) eines gekochten Schweine-Kinnbacken und 1 Unze vom

Nr. 29

When a horse is overheated

Take ½ pint of flax seed oil
½ pint of hogs lard

Mix it together, give it to the horse and wash him with fresh water.

Nr. 30

For a swelling

Take argentite [Ag_2S] and an equal amount of good vinegar. Mix them and allow the mixture to stand for one hour. Then add sweet oil until the mixture is fluid. Smear the preparation on the swollen part.

Nr. 31

To make an excellent salve that heals a wound that may be caused by the saddle, the horse collar or perhaps something else

Take 2 ounces of fat from a cooked hog jaw and one ounce of the best gunpowder. Make the powder very fine and mix it with the fat. Use it morning and evening.

— 17 —

besten Schießpulver. Mache das Pulver recht fein und mische es mit dem Fett. Gebrauche es Morgens und Abends.

Nro. 32.

Das Blut zu stillen.

Nimm harten Ruß aus einem Schornsteine, mache ihn recht fein und mische ihn mit Whiskey, bis es eine Salbe gibt. Binde es auf die Wunde.

Nro. 33.

Wenn ein Pferd krank ist und man seine Krankheit nicht kennt oder versteht.

Gib dem Pferde Morgens 2 Unzen Borax in dem Futter; den andern Morgen dieselbe Quantität Borax mit 2 Unzen Nelkenpfeffer (alspice); den dritten Morgen gib ihm nur 2 Unzen Nelkenpfeffer; den vierten Morgen gib ihm 46 Gräne Calomel und alsdann laß es zur Ader.

Nro. 34.

Wenn ein Pferd nicht fressen will.

Nimm 1 Peint Wein und ½ Unze Teufelsdreck (asafoetida), und koche es ein wenig. Gib es dem Pferde lauwarm.

B

Nr. 32

To stop bleeding

Take hard soot from the chimney and pulverize it. Mix this with whiskey until it has the consistency of a salve. Bind it on the wound.

Nr. 33

If a horse is sick and one does not recognize the sickness or understand it

Give the horse two ounces of borax in his fodder in the morning. On the second morning, give him the same quantity of borax and two ounces of allspice. On the third morning give him only two 2 ounces of allspice. On the fourth morning, give him forty-six grains of calomel and then bleed him.

Nr. 34

If a horse will not eat

Take one pint of wine and one-half ounce of asafetida and cook it a little. Give this, lukewarm, to the horse.

— 18 —

Nro. 35.

Wenn ein Pferd sehr krank ist, zu erfahren ob es wieder aufkommt oder nicht.

Nimm ein Tschill von Gewürzholzbeeren, mache sie fein, gieße ein Peint Wein und ein Peint Wasser auf das Pulver und tränke das Pferd mit der Mischung; bleibt es bei ihm, so kommt es davon, wenn nicht, so stirbt es.

Nro. 36.

Für geschwollene Beine.

Nimm gebrannten Lehm aus einem Backofen, mache ihn fein und mische ihn mit Essig und Salz, bis er zur Salbe wird; hievon schmiere auf ein weißes wollenes Tuch und binde es um den geschwollenen Theil; lasse es 24 Stunden drauf und dann erneure es wieder, und so verfahre 3 oder 4 Tage lang, so wird das Pferd curirt seyn.

Nro. 37.

Ein Blasenpflaster für ein Pferd zu machen.

Nimm Weizenmehl, Honig, Eierweiß und Wein; schlage alles zusammen und wende es an.

Nr. 35

To determine if a very sick horse will survive or not

Take a gill of Jamaica Pepper and pulverize it. Pour a pint of wine and a pint of water over the powder then water the horse with this mixture. If he retains it, he will recover and if not he will die.

Nr. 36

For swollen legs

Take burned clay out of a bake oven and pulverize it. Mix the powder with vinegar and salt until it is like a salve. Smear this on a white woolen cloth and bind it around the swollen part. Leave it on for twenty-four hours and then renew it. Proceed in this way for three to four days and then the horse will be cured.

Nr. 37

To make a blasenpflaster a plaster that will absorb a quantity of liquid for a horse

Take flour, honey, egg white and wine. Beat these all together and use it.

— 19 —

Nro. 38.

Zu verhindern, daß die Fliegen die Pferde quälen.

Nimm eine Handvoll Knoblauch, schneide ihn fein, und ebenso viel Hammelsfett, schmelze es und mische den Knoblauch unter das Fett. Dieses Gemisch reibe oberflächlich übers Pferd.

Nro. 39.

Wenn eine Stute nicht empfängt.

Gib ihr 40 Tropfen Canthariodes-Tinktur, 12 Stunden ehe sie zum Hengst gethan wird.

Nro. 40.

Die Läuse zu zerstören.

Nimm ½ Unze Tabacks-Blätter, ½ Unze Gewürzholzbeeren pulverisirt, 1 Unze Quecksilber, 1½ Unze Lorbeeröl; mische alles zusammen. Schmiere hiemit die beschädigten Theile. Oder schmiere davon auf ein wollenes Tuch und binde es um des Thieres Hals herum.—Leinöl angewendet ist auch wirksam.

Nr. 38

To prevent flies from tormenting a horse

Take a handful of garlic and cut it fine. Take an equal quantity of mutton fat, melt it and mix the garlic under the melted fat. This mixture is rubbed over the surface of the horse.

Nr. 39

If a mare will not conceive

Give her forty drops of Cantharides Tincture [Spanish Fly] twelve hours before presenting the stallion to her.

Nr. 40

To destroy lice

Take one-half ounce of tobacco leaves, one-half ounce of pulverized Jamaica pepper, one ounce of quick silver and one and one-half ounces laurel oil and mix everything together. Smear the affected part with the mixture or smear some on a woolen cloth and tie it around the neck of the animal. The use of linseed oil is also effective.

— 20 —

Nro. 41.

Wenn ein Pferd sehr krank ist in den Eingeweiden,

verursacht durch Trinken kalten Wassers in einem erhitzten Zustande. Man hört ein Gerumpel in seinem Leibe, es legt sich plötzlich, steht wieder auf und will nicht fressen.

Nimm 2 Drachmen Gewürzholzbeeren
" 1 " Bockshorn (fenugreek)
" 1 " schwarzen Pfeffer
" 1 " Zitwer (zedoary)
" 1 " Gewürznelken
" 1 Skrupel Saffran.

Pulverisire alles, schütte ein Peint Wein dazu und koche es einige Minuten.—Gib es auf einmal.—Wenn nöthig, wiederhole es in 12 Stunden.

Nro. 42.

Für den Engerling (bots).

Nimm 8 Unzen Bienenwachs
" 8 " Hammelsfett
" 8 " Hutzucker. Thue alles in eine Quart frische Milch und mache es warm bis alles aufgelöst ist.—Gib es all auf einmal.

In 2 Stunden darauf gib ein Abführungsmittel.

Nr. 41

Sick in the bowels

If a horse is very sick in the bowels, and if this is caused by drinking cold water in a heated condition, and if one hears a continuous rumbling in his body, and the horse lies down suddenly, stands up again and will not eat:

Take 2 drams of Jamaican pepper
1 dram of fenugreek [Trigonella foenumgraecum]
1 dram of black pepper
1 dram of zedoary [*Curcuma zedoary*, white tumeric]
1 dram of parsley
1 pinch of saffron

Pulverize the ingredients and dust the powder into a pint of wine and cook a few minutes. Give it all at one time. If necessary, repeat in twelve hours.

Nr. 42

For bots

Take 8 ounces of beeswax
8 ounces of mutton fat
8 ounces of loaf sugar

Put everything into a quart of fresh milk and warm it until it is all dissolved. Give it all at once. In two hours give a purgative.

— 21 —

Nro. 43.

Ein vortreffliches Pferdepulver zu machen.

Nimm 1 Unze Spießglas (Antimony)
" 2 " Weinsteinrahm
" 2 " Harz (rosin)
" 2 " Schwefelblüthe
" 2 " Salpeter
" 2 " Bockshorn (fenugreek)
Gib jeden Tag einen Eßlöffel voll bis es all ist.

Nro. 44.

Für den Founder.

Nimm 1 Peint Schmierseife und 7 Hühnereier; schlage es wohl durch einander und gib es auf einmal.

Nro. 45.

Der Polibel und die Fistel.

Nimm einen Klumpen gewöhnliches Salz von der Größe eines Hühnereis und eben soviel harte Seife: nimm eine Quantität palk root und koche sie besonders, bis es ein Syrup wird, (in

Nr. 43

To make an excellent horse powder

Take 1 ounce of antimony
2 ounces of cream of tartar
2 ounces of rosin
2 ounces of flowers of sulfur
2 ounces of saltpeter
2 ounces of fenugreek
[*Trigonella foenuaecumgraecum*]

Every day give a tablespoonful until it is all gone.

Nr. 44

For the founder [laminitis]

Take one pint of soft soap and seven hen's eggs; beat them all together and give it as one dose.

Nr. 45

The polibel [poll evil] and the fistula

Take a clump of ordinary salt about the size of a hen's egg and a like amount of hand soap. Take a quantity of Palk root [Poke weed] and cook it separately until it becomes a syrup [make a pint], then mix in the salt and the soap so that it forms a ball. Wash the afflicted place every morning for a week and it will effect a cure.

— 22 —

Quantität 1 Peint); alsdann mische das Salz und die Seife darunter, so daß es einen Ballen macht. Wasche den Platz jeden Morgen für eine Woche lang, so wird eine Cur bewirkt.

Nro. 46.

Das Haar wachsen zu machen.

Brenne grüne Wallnüsse zu Pulver, mische das Pulver mit Honig, Bäumöl und Wein, und schmiere alsdann den Ort damit.

Nro. 47.

Für Ueberbeine (wens) an irgend einem Theile des Körpers.

Zuerst brenne sie mit einem glühenden Eisen, alsdann heile es mit dem Pulver von Honig und Kalk.—Es heilt gleich.

Nro. 48.

Für den Schwären (**Botch**) oder irgend ein Geschwür.

Nimm ein Stück mit Alaun zubereiteres Leder so groß als das Geschwür, schmiere Schuhmacher-

Nr. 46

To make hair grow

Burn green walnuts to a powder, mix the powder with honey, olive oil and wine and then smear the spot with the mixture.

Nr. 47

For Ueberbeine (wens) on nearly any part of the body

First burn it with a glowing iron then heal the burn with a powder of honey and chalk. It heals well.

Nr. 48

For the Schwaeren (botch) [bots] or any swelling

Take a piece of leather as large as the swelling, which has been dressed with alum, and smear it with shoemaker's wax. Lay this prepared leather on the swelling until it is ripe. When it is ripe open it and wash the wound with alum water. Then smear it with a salve called Egyptiacum [contains alum, basic copper acetate, corrosive sublimate] whereby it is soon healed.

— 23 —

Wax darauf und lege es auf das Geschwür, so wird es reif. Wann es reif geworden ist, öffne es, wasche die Wunde mit Alaunwasser aus und schmiere sie mit der Salbe genannt Egyptiacum, wodurch sie bald heilt.

Nro. 49.

Für den Krebs oder wunde Stelle an irgend einem Theile des Körpers.

Koche eine Quantität palk root in einer Quart Wasser bis zu einem halben Peint; alsdann nimm 6 Unzen Schmalz, 1 Tschill Theer (tar) und 1 Unze Schwefelblumen, koche alles zusammen bis das Wasser verkocht ist und gebrauche es als eine Salbe für einigen heftigen Krebs oder wunde Stelle.

Nro. 50.

Für den Strengel.

Laß das Pferd unter der Zunge zur Ader, und dämpfe es mit einer Abkochung von Kamillen, und mache einen Umschlag von Kleie, Essig, Salz und Schmalz. Es wird bald heilen.

Nr. 49

For cancer or a wound on any place on the body

Cook a quantity of Palk root [Poke weed] in a quart of water until the volume is reduced to a half pint. Then take six ounces of lard, one gill of tar, one ounce of flowers of sulfur and cook everything together until the water is all removed. Use this as a salve for severe cancer or sore.

Nr. 50

For strengel [an infection of lymph nodes]

Bleed the horse under his tongue and dampen it with decoction of camomile [*Anthemis nobilis*], Make a dressing of clay, vinegar, salt and lard. It will soon heal.

— 24 —

Nro. 51.

Für den Hoden (Stone).

Nimm ½ Unze Salpeter, eine gute Wurzel Meerrettig fein gerieben, thue es in eine Quart Wein oder klaren Seider und thue 6 fein gestoßene Eierschalen hinzu. Lasse es 24 Stunden stehen, alsdann gib es dem Pferde; wenn nöthig, kannst du es auch früher geben.

Nro. 52.

Für den Engerling (bots).

Nimm ½ Peint Urin
" 1 Tschill Rum
" 1 großen Eßlöffel voll Pfeffer
" 1 " " " Schießpulver.

Schüttele es wohl durch einander und schütte es dem Pferde ein. — Es ist eine absolute Cur.

Nro. 53.

Ein Blasenpflaster.

Nimm 2 Unzen Nervensalbe
" 2 " Eibisch (marshmallow)

Nr. 51

For stones

Take one-half ounce of saltpeter and a finely grated good root of horseradish and put this in a quart of wine or clear cider. Then add six finely pulverized egg-shells. Let it stand for twenty-four hours and give it to the horse. If necessary you can repeat it.

Nr. 52

For Engerling (bots)

Take ½ pint of urine
1 gill of rum
1 large tablespoonful of pepper
1 large tablespoonful of gunpowder

Mix thoroughly by shaking well and sprinkle it on the horse. It is an absolute cure.

Nr. 53

A blasenpflaster

Take 2 ounces of Nerve salve
[*ungeuentum rosimarini compositum*]
2 ounces of Marshmallow
1 ounce of quick silver
1 ounce of oil of turpentine
1 ½ drachem of Spanish Fly
1 drachem of Sublimate [Sublimate of Mercury]
2 drachem of Organum [*Organum syriacum*]

Very good.

— 25 —

" 1 " Quecksilber
" 1 " Venice Terpentinöl
" 1½ Drachmen pulverisirte spanische Mücken
" 1 " Sublimat
" 2 " Origanum.
Sehr gut.

Nro. 54.

Um Geschwüre zur Reife zu bringen.

Zerstoße Pappelwurzeln und weiße Lilienwurzeln, koche sie in Milch, verdicke es mit Leinmehl. —Applizire es Umschlagsweise.

Nro. 55.

Für ein krebsartiges Geschwür an den Füßen.

Nimm Kuhfladen, Theer und Schmalz, mache einen Umschlag davon so heiß als möglich, doch so daß es nicht brennt, und binde denselben um den Huf herum.

Nro. 56.

Für gedrückte Schultern.

Nimm ½ Peint Rum und ein Stück harte Seife, mache einen Schaum daraus und wasche

C

Nr. 54

To bring a swelling to a head

Crush by beating Poplar roots and white lily roots, cook them in milk and thicken with linseed meal. Apply as a dressing.

Nr. 55

For a cancer-like swelling on the foot

Take cow dung, tar and lard and make a dressing from the mixture as hot as possible, however not so hot that it burns. Bind the dressing around the hoof.

Nr. 56

For pinched shoulder

Take one-half pint of rum and a piece of hard soap, make a froth with this and wash the shoulder. Allow it to harden and it will heal the shoulder. Rattlesnake fat serves the same purpose.

damit die Schultern; es härtet und heilt sie. Klapperschlangenfett thut dieselben Dienste.

Nro. 57.

Für den Anfang von einer Fistel oder Polibel.

Nimm Rainfarn (tansy), Wermuth und assesmart, zerstoße alles und thue kalt Wasser darauf dann thue es in ein Säckchen, lege es auf die beschädigte Stelle, lasse es 2 Stunden darauf, alsdann nimm es ab und vergrabe es unter die Wurzel einer der obigen Kräuter. Sobald es fault, wird der Schaden sich heben und vergehen. Wo diese Schäden hartnäckig sind ist Guaiacum Oehl oder Palmöl sehr gut, die Geschwulst zu lindern.

Nro. 58.

Für Gift.

Raute (rue) in frische Milch gekocht und zum Trinken gegeben ist ein sehr gutes Gegengift.

Nro. 59.

Für das Gelbe Wasser.

Nimm 2 Unzen Spießglas (antimony)
" 2 " geläuterter Salpeter

Nr. 57

For a beginning fistula or polibel [poll evil]

Take Tansy, Wormwood and Assesmart [Smartweed], crush them and add cold water. Place them in a small sack and lay it on the afflicted place. Leave it on for two hours and then remove it and bury it under the roots of the plants mentioned above. As soon as it rots, the affliction will be relieved and disappear. When the affliction is stubborn, Guaiacum Oil [oil from *Guaicum officinale*] or Palm oil is very good to alleviate the swelling.

Nr. 58

For poisoning

Rue [*Ruta graveolens*] cooked in fresh milk and given to drink is a very good antidote.

Nr. 59

For dirt malanders

Take 2 ounces of antimony stibnite
2 ounces of purified saltpeter
2 ounces of flowers of sulfur
2 ounces of cream of tartar

First mix the antimony and saltpeter then add the flowers of sulfur and cream of tartar. Give the horse as much as can be put on a penny three times a day. The above is the best cure to come before the public.

— 27 —

„ 2 „ Schwefelblüthe
„ 2 „ Weinsteinrahm.

Zuerst mische das Spießglas und den Salpeter, alsdann thue die Schwefelblüthe und den Weinsteinrahm dazu.

Gib dem Pferd so viel als auf einem Cent liegen bleibt, dreimal des Tags. Obiges ist die beste Cur, die je vor das Publikum gekommen.

Nro. 60.

Eine gewisse Cur für die Sweeny.

Nimm schimmligen Speck, schneide ihn fein und lasse das Fett aus, alsdann thue 2 Theetassen voll feines Salz und 3 frische Eier zu einem halben Peint Schmalz und rühre es wohl durch einander, bis es kalt ist.—Mit dieser Salbe schmiere den beschädigten Theil den dritten, fünften und siebenten Tag nach dem neuen Monde. Es schlägt nie fehl.

Nro. 61.

Für den Engerling oder Würmer.

Nimm 1 Tschill Rum und 2 Unzen Pilgrimssalbe, schüttele es wohl durch einander und gib es dem Pferd. Es hilft gleich.

Nr. 60

A certain cure for the Sweeney [atrophy of the shoulder muscles]

Take moldy lard cut it into small pieces and melt the fat. Add two teaspoonfuls of fine salt and three fresh eggs. Add this warm mixture to a half pint of mutton fat and stir well until it is cold. Smear this salve on the afflicted part the third, fifth and seventh day after the new moon. It never fails.

Nr. 61

For bots or worms

Take one shill of rum and two ounces of Pilgrims Salve, mix thoroughly by shaking and give it to the horse. It helps immediately. [Pilgrims salve is a vulgar early nineteenth-century slang term for a paste made from moist human excrement.]

— 28 —

Nro. 62.

Für die Räude.

Löse 6 Unzen Kalkstein in 3 Quart starkem Bier auf und gib es dem Pferd auf zweimal, nämlich das zweitemal nach 2 Tagen. Es heilt gewiß.

Nro. 63.

Eine gewisse Cur für die Flechsenverletzung.

Nimm ein Peint Weinhefen, stelle sie übers Feuer, dann nimm etwas Wanderde, worin kein Kalk ist, und thue es dazu und koche es bis zur Dickung einer Salbe und klappe es heiß auf die Beschädigung.

Nro. 64.

Für spröde Hufen.

Nimm Schweinefett, Hundefett und Terpentin, von jedem gleichviel, mische alles wohl zusammen, und schmiere damit die Hufen. Hundefett ist vortrefflich für spröde Hufen.

Nr. 62

For mange

Dissolve six ounces of limestone in three quarts of strong beer and give it to the horse twice. The second time two days after the first. It certainly helps.

Nr. 63

A certain cure for an injured tendon

Take a pint of wine yeast and place it over the fire. Take some Wanderde [clay] that contains no lime and add it to the yeast. Cook the mixture until it thickens to a salve and clap it hot over the affliction.

Nr. 64

For brittle hoofs

Take equal amounts of lard, dog's fat and turpentine and mix them together. Smear this mixture on the hoof. Dog fat is excellent for brittle hoofs.

— 29 —

Nro. 65.

Für die Räude.

Laß am Halse zur Ader ein= oder zweimal, reiße mit dem Krämpelkamm den Schorf ab, und nimm alsdann Theer (tar), Terpentin und Leinöl, so viel als du für gut ansiehst, menge es wohl durcheinander und schmiere davon heiß (doch so daß es nicht brennt) auf die beschädigten Theile. Ein einziges Mal geschmiert bewirkt eine gewisse Cur.

N. B. Reinige den Sattel und Kummet gut, ehe du sie bei einem andern Pferde gebrauchst, denn die Krankheit ist ansteckend.

Nro. 66.

Für wehe Augen, oder Blindheit, wo die Ballen gesund sind.

Nimm ein Ei und mache oben ein Loch hinein und lasse die Hälfte herauslaufen, dann fülle es mit wohl gemischten gleichen Theilen von Salz und Ingber, wickele es in ein nasses Tuch ein, thue es ins Feuer und röste es recht hart; dann nimm es heraus und mache es zu Pulver.—Vor der Application wasche das Auge mit dem Wasser des Augentrosts und dem Saft von gemahle=

Nr. 65

For the mange

Bleed the neck vein once or twice. Scrape off the mange scab with an iron comb and then take as much as you require of tar, turpentine and linseed oil. Mix the ingredients thoroughly and smear the hot—but not so hot that it burns—mixture on the affected part. A single application will produce a certain cure.

Note: Clean the saddle and horse collar thoroughly before using them on another horse, because the disease is contagious.

Nr. 66

For sore eyes or blindness where the eyeballs are sound

Make a hole in the shell of an egg and let half of the contents run out. Then fill the egg with well-mixed equal parts of salt and ginger, wrap it in a moist cloth and heat it very strongly in the fire. Remove it from the fire and pulverize it. Before the application, wash the eye with the water of Eye Bright [an herb of the figwort genus] and the sap of ground-up ivy. After washing, blow the powder into the eye using the shaft of a feather.

— 30 —

nem Epheu und blase alsdann mit einem Federkeile das Pulver hinein.

Nro. 67.

Eine bewährte Cur für Blindheit.

Nimm Vermillion, Betonie und Lavendel, stoße alles in einem Mörser, bis es zu einem dicken Teig oder Salbe wird; mache es in Kuchen von $\frac{3}{4}$ Zoll im Durchmesser; trockne sie; dann thue sie in einem Hafen oder Schüssel auf Kohlen, decke sie mit einem Trichter zu und laß den Rauch in seine Nasenlöcher gehen; dies thue Morgens und Abends. Jedesmal, wann du es räucherst, wasche seine Augen mit dem Wasser des Augentrostes und dem Saft vom gemahlenen Epheu.

Nro. 68.

Für den Krebs im Auge.

Ziehe Blut an der Ader am Schlafe, dann nimm Kupferwasser (copperas) und gebrannten Alaun, von jedem gleichviel; backe es zusammen auf einem Stein oder Eisen, mache es dann zu Pulver und setze so viel Honig zu, bis daß es eine Salbe wird. Nimm eine Feder und schmiere damit die wunde Stelle.

Es wird gewißlich den Kanker heilen.

Nr. 67

A true cure for blindness

Take vermillion, bentonite and lavender and grind them in a mortar until they become a thick paste or salve. Form this paste into a cookie three-quarter inches in diameter, dry it and place it in a jar or dish on the coals. Cover it with a funnel and let the smoke go into the horse's nostrils. Do this in the morning and the evening. Every time you smoke the horse, wash his eyes with water of Eye Bright and the sap of ground-up ivy.

Nr. 68

For a canker in the eye

Bleed the horse during sleep, then take copperas [a green hydrated ferrous sulfate] and burnt alum in equal amounts and bake them together on a stone or iron plate. Pulverize this mixture and add sufficient honey until it forms a salve. Take a feather and smear this salve on the wounded place.

It certainly will heal the canker.

— 31 —

Nro. 69.

Für die Windgalle.

Raßiere die Haare ab, dann kriege die innere Rinde der weißen Wallnuß,—klappe sie auf die Galle und binde sie darauf, lasse es 24 Stunden darauf; während dieser Zeit aber solltest du davon in frischem Wasser kochen und davon auf die Galle schütten, um zu verhindern daß die Rinde trocken wird; nach 24 Stunden nimm die Rinde weg und schmiere den Platz mit frischer Butter oder Schweinefett. Es wirkt mit Erfolg.

Nro. 70.

Für steife oder verletzte Flechsen.

Nimm ein Pfund schwarze Seife und koche sie in einer Quart Ael (ale) bis zur Dicke einer gewöhnlichen Salbe. Schmiere damit die Flechsen und Gelenke, so werden sie geschmeidig werden und ihre gehörige Ausdehnung bekommen, obschon sie zuvor noch so zusammen geschrumpft waren.

Nro. 71.

Für eine Verrenkung in der Fessel.

Ein Pflaster von Kronenseife und Brändy heiß angewendet ist sehr gut. Halte das Pferd aus

Nr. 69

For the windgall

First shave the hair from the gall then take the inner bark from the white walnut, clap it on the gall and bind it fast. Leave the bark in place for twenty-four hours. During this time cook some fresh water and pour this over the gall in order to prevent the bark from becoming dry. After 24 hours, remove the bark and smear the place with fresh butter or lard. It will be successful.

Nr. 70

For stiff or injured tendons

Cook a pound of black soap in a quart of ale until it attains the consistency of ordinary salve. Smear the tendons and joint with this salve and they will become pliant and return to their proper size even though they were previously shriveled.

Nr. 71

For the dislocation of the fetlock

The use of a hot plaster of Crown Soap [a type of very high quality soap] and brandy is very good. Keep the horse out of water for a week or so until you see that the horse can function properly again.

— 32 —

dem Wasser eine Woche lang darauf, bis du siehst daß es wieder gut gehen kann.

Die obige Seife und Brändy ist eine absolute Cur für Verrenkung oder Geschwulst, sey diese so hart wie ein Knochen. Zuerst schmiere mit Terpentinöl und Bier und nach einem oder zwei Tagen applizire die Seife und Brändy. Es wird eine baldige Cur bewirken.

Nro. 72.

Für eine Entzündung der Drüsen zwischen den Kinnbacken und dem Halse, genannt die Feifel (vives).

Nimm einen Theelöffel voll schwarzen Pfeffer, einen Eßlöffel voll Schweinefett, den Saft von einer Handvoll Raute und 2 Löffel voll guten Essig; mische alles zusammen und thue es gleich vertheilt in die Ohren des Pferdes, binde sie mit 2 platten Schnüren zu und mache daß die Medizin hinunter geht; alsdann ziehe Blut an den Hals- und Schlafadern.

Nro. 73.

Für den Nierengries (gravel).

Nimm 2 Zwiebeln und lasse sie in Wein einige Zeit liegen. Gib es dem Pferd, so wird es gleich Linderung bekommen.

The above soap and brandy is an absolute cure for dislocation or swelling, even if it is as hard as bone. First smear it with turpentine and beer and then after one or two days apply the soap and brandy. This will quickly effect a cure.

Nr. 72

For an inflammation of the glands between the jaw bone and the neck, called the vives

Mix together a teaspoonful of lard, the sap from a handful of rue and two spoonfuls of good vinegar. Apply equal parts in the ears of the horse and bind them with two flat straps. See that the medicine goes down then draw blood from the neck and temporal veins.

Nr. 73

For kidney stones (gravel)

Take two onions and let them stand in wine for a time. Give it to the horse and it will have immediate relief.

It helps the horse to immediately pass the grits, sand, stone and tartrate material.

— 33 —

Es hilft dem Pferd sogleich und schafft den Gries, Sand, Stein und die weinsteinartige Materie fort.

Nro. 74.

Für die tolle Krätze.

Zuerst lasse es am Halse zur Ader, dann koche starke Lauge und Essig mit Schießpulver und Kupferwasser; mache es recht stark, befestige ein Tuch an einen Stecken und wasche die wunden Stellen. Es schlägt nie fehl.

Nro. 75.

Auslaufende Drüsen.

Zuerst bemerke, wenn du dem Pferde Hafer geben willst, daß du zuvor etwas Honig unter dieselbe mischest und mit deinen Händen gut durcheinander reibest; hiemit fahre fort bis das Auslaufen aus der Nase aufhört. Dies ist eins der gewissesten Mittel, denn es vertreibt allen Schleim und Galle, reinigt den Kopf, das Gehirn und Blut, zertheilt böse Feuchtigkeiten, verursacht gute Verdauung und befreit das Pferd von Drüsen, Verkältung, Gift und Auslaufen aus der Nase.

Nr. 74

For frantic scratching [mange]

First bleed the neck vein. Then cook strong lye and vinegar with gunpowder and Kupferwasser [copper water, copper sulfate solution] until concentrated. Fasten a cloth to a stick and wash the afflicted spot with the mixture. It is never amiss.

Nr. 75

Discharging glands

Before giving the horse his oats, mix some honey with the oats and rub them together with your hands. Then walk the horse around until his nasal discharge stops. This is one of the best known agents to expel all mucus and bile, purify the head, brain, and blood. It disperses bad dampness, brings about good digestion and frees the horse from glands, chills, poison and discharges from the nose.

Nro. 76.

Für die Drüsen.

Nimm frischen Urin und starken weißen Weinessig, von jedem ein halbes Peint, 3 Eßlöffel voll Senfsamen, diesen mische mit Essig, dann thue den Urin und Essig zum Senf und rühre sie wohl zusammen; ferner nimm eine gleiche Quantität Theer (tar) und Baysalz, so viel als hinreichend seyn mag, und mische es wohl zusammen und bringe 1½ Tschills bei.

Nachdem diese Dinge zubereitet sind, so halte das Pferd über Nacht sparsam im Futter und den nächsten Morgen reite es bis es recht schwitzt, dann gib ihm das Salz und Theer, wie oben vorgeschrieben, und sobald als es dieses genommen hat, so gib ihm mit einem Horn oben besagtes Getränk, gemacht von frischem Urin, Essig und Senf, alle zum Maul hinein, ausgenommen zwei kleine Hörner voll, die ihm in die Nasenlöcher geschüttet werden müssen; nachdem es auch dieses genommen hat so reite es wieder wie zuvor, stelle es auf, bedecke es wohl und mache eine gute Streu; lasse es mit dem Gebiß stehen bis 4 Uhr; alsdann nimm ihm das Gebiß ab, gib ihm warmes Futter (mash), und behandele es in allem, so wie man mit Pferden zu thun pflegt, die Medizin nehmen; gib ihm diese Medizin oder Getränk alle 2 Tage, wenn es stark ist; ist es aber schwach, alle 3 oder 4 Tage.

Nr. 76

For the glands

Use a half pint of fresh urine and a half pint of strong white wine vinegar. Take three tablespoons of mustard seed and mix it with some of the vinegar. Then add the urine and the remaining vinegar to the mustard and mix by stirring thoroughly. Take a like amount of tar and as much bay salt as may be necessary and thoroughly mix these together. Use one and one-half gills.

After these things are prepared, keep the horse on sparse feed overnight. The next morning ride him until he is perspiring heavily and then give him the salt and tar as described above. As soon as he has taken this, give him a horn of the drink mentioned above made from urine, vinegar and mustard, all by mouth except for two small horns-full that must be poured into his nostrils. After this is done ride him again as previously. Then cover him well and make a good bed of straw. Let him remain four hours with a bit and then remove the bit and give him warm mash. Treat him in every way like a horse taking medicine. Give the horse this medicine or drink for two days if it is strong for three or four days if it is weak.

This is an infallible cure if it is applied three or four times and administered in the correct fashion, even if the horse is exhausted.

— 35 —

Dies ist eine unfehlbare Cur, wenn es 3 oder 4 Mal und zwar rechter Art gegeben wird; obgleich das Pferd ziemlich erschöpft wäre.

Nro. 77.

Leberkrankheit, als Entzündung, Hinderungen und Auszehrung.

Die Leber, welche das Gefäß des Bluts ist, ist vielen Krankheiten unterworfen, je nachdem eine Verwirrung des Bluts stattfindet. Die Zeichen sind, ein stinkender Athem und ein natürliches Hinblicken nach seinem Bauche.

Die Cur ist, Aristolochia longa in Springwasser gekocht, bis das Wasser halb eingekocht ist; hievon laß das Pferd beständig trinken. Es heilt alle Uebel der Leber.

Nro. 78.

Gallenkrankheit, besonders die Gelbsucht.

Von dem Ueberfließen der Galle entspringen viele tödtliche Krankheiten, besonders die Gelbsucht, welches eine sehr ermattende Krankheit ist und tödtlich ausfällt, wenn nicht zeitige Hilfsmittel angewendet werden. Die Zeichen sind, daß die Au-

Nr. 77

Liver disease such as inflammation, obstructions and wasting away

The liver, the container of the blood, is subjected to many illnesses, according to what disruption of the blood takes place. The symptoms are a stinking breath and the condition of the horse's abdomen. The cure is *Aristolochia longa* [long root or birthwort], cooked in spring water until the volume is decreased to one half. Then let the horse drink it straight down. It heals all evils of the liver.

Nr. 78

Bilious sickness, especially jaundice

Many deadly diseases arise from the overflow of bile, especially jaundice. Jaundice is a very exhausting disease with fatal consequences if remedial medicine is not administered in time.

The signs are that the eyes and skin mainly under the upper lip near the front teeth become yellow. A sudden debilitating collapse and general sweating over the whole body accompany these signs. The cure is bleeding the neck or mouth vein or under the eyes. Then dry and pulverize a small amount of saffron [dried anthers of *Crocus sativus*]. Mix this powder with sweet butter and form it into pills. Give these pills to the horse for three mornings. Make his drink warm and sprinkle his hay with water before you give it to him.

— 36 —

gen und Haut gelb werden, hauptsächlich unter der Oberlippe nahe den Vorderzähnen, ein plötzliches und ermattendes Niederfallen und ein allgemeiner Schweiß über den ganzen Körper. Die Cur ist, erstens, ein Aderlaß am Halse, oder Maul, oder unter den Augen, dann nimm ein wenig Saffran und trockene und mache es zu Pulver, mische es mit süßer Butter und mache Pillen daraus, gib es dem Pferde für 3 Morgen zusammen, mache sein Getränk warm und besprenge das Heu mit Wasser, ehe du es ihm gibst.

Nro. 79.

Für eine Verrenkung an der Fessel.

Nimm Biersatz, Hühnerdreck, Nervenöl und frisches Fett, darin nie Salz war, mache einen Umschlag davon und lege ihn darauf; dies ist vortrefflich für eine Verrenkung an der Fessel oder Hufhaar, und heilt bald.

Nro. 80.

Allgemeiner Krampf oder Erschütterung der Flechsen.

Krämpfe sind ein Zusammenziehen der Flechsen irgend eines Glieds; Erschütterungen aber

Nr. 79

For dislocation of the fetlock joint

Make a poultice from Biersass [sediment in beer brewing vats], chicken dirt, Nervenoel [a patent remedy containing an essential oil from the mint family] and fresh fat that contains no salt and place it on the affected part. This is poultice is excellent for a dislocated fettock joint or fettock. It heals them quickly.

Nr. 80

General cramps or shock of the tendon

Cramps are the contraction of the tendons of some limbs but 'shocking' is if the body from head to foot is generally contracted or stiffened.

The cure for both conditions is to first rub the contracted limb with vinegar and ordinary oil and then completely cover it with wet hay or a woolen cloth. This agent rapidly heals both.

sind, wenn der Körper vom Kopf an bis zum äußersten Theile, gemeiniglich zusammengezogen oder steif ist.

Die Cur für beide ist erstens, reibe das zusammengezogene Glied mit Essig und ordinärem Oel und dann bedecke es gänzlich mit nassem Heu oder mit wollenen Tüchern, beides ist ein geschwindes Heilmittel.

Nro. 81.

Schmerzen in den Nieren, Hod 2c.

Alle diese Krankheiten entstehen aus einer Ursache, nämlich aus der Sammlung von Sand oder sonst harter Materie in den Nieren, weil dadurch die Röhre des Urins verstopft wird. Die Zeichen sind, daß ein Pferd öfters sich heftig anstrengt um zu pissen, kann aber nicht; die Cur ist, nimm eine Handvoll Frauenhaar und lasse sie in einer Quart starkem Ael (ale) über Nacht stehen, und gib es dann dem Pferde jeden Morgen zu trinken, bis es curirt ist. Es bricht irgend einen Stein in einem Pferde.

Nro. 82.

Für den Blutspath oder irgend eine andere unnatürliche Geschwulst.

Dies sind Keulen oder weiche runde Geschwülste, das erste ist von don dem hintern innern Ge-

Nr. 81

Pain in the kidneys, testicles, etc.

All these diseases result from one origin, namely an accumulation of sand or otherwise hard material in the kidney and through this the ureters become clogged. The aflicted horse often, very strongly, strains to urinate without success. The cure is to take a handful of Maidenhair and let it stand overnight in a quart of strong ale and then give it to the horse to drink every morning until he is cured. It breaks up any stone in a horse.

Nr. 82

For the blutspath [blood spavin] or any other unnatural swelling

These are club-shaped or soft round swellings that originate from the back of the inside joint below the thigh. They are soft and very sore. The cure is to first bind the vein above the swelling and open the vein only below the swelling and draw blood. Then bind the vein both above and below the swelling and slit the vein. Next, take linseeds, crush them fine in a mortar, mix it together with fresh cow dung, heat the mixture in a pan and place it on the swelling. When this swelling ruptures and drains, heal it with a pitch plaster. The horse will never again be plagued with this. If the swelling is the result of a sprain or a bruise, take tar, melt it and smear it on the wounded place. Also hold a hot iron close to it in order to make the grease run into the wound. Then bind the wound up with a cloth and the swelling will be healed successfully.

— 38 —

lenke unter dem Dickbeine; sie sind weich und sehr wund. Die Cur ist also: zuerst binde die Ader oben zu, und öffne sie nur von unten und ziehe Blut, dann binde sie fest zu an beiden Seiten und schlitze die Ader entzwei; dann nimm Leinsamen und stoße es in einem Mörser fein, mische es zusammen mit frischen Kuhfladen, mache es heiß in einer Pfanne und thue es nur auf die Geschwulst; wenn dieselbe aufbricht und ausläuft, so heile es mit einem Pflaster von Pech— das Pferd wird nie wieder damit geplagt seyn. Wenn die Geschwulst durch eine Verrenkung oder Quetschung kommt, so nimm Pechschmalz, schmelze es und schmiere damit die wunde Stelle, auch halte ein heißes Eisen nahe bei, um das Schmalz recht eindringen zu machen, dann verbinde es mit einem leinen Tuch, so wird die Geschwulst gelindert werden.

Nro. 83.

Irgend ein gebrochenes inwendiges Glied oder Ader wieder zu verbinden.

Nimm Drachen-Saffran und die Frucht der Fichte, Eidotter, mische es zusammen mit Wein und Oel; dieses gib dem Pferd, so heilt jedes inwendige Glied, oder gebrochene Ader.

Nr. 83

To mend any internal organ or broken vein

Take Drachen-Saffran [a mixture of Dragon Blood and Saffron], egg yolks and mix these together with wine and oil. Give the mixture to the horse and it will heal any internal organ or broken vein. [Dragon's blood is a bright red resin obtained from the juice of a number of distinct plant genera such as *Croton*, *Dracaena*, *Daemonorops*, *Calamus rotang* and *Pterocarpus*.]

— 39 —

Nro. 84.

Für die Hitze im Maul.

Mache mit der Lanze einen Schnitt in die obere Lippe und wasche es mit Essig und Salz zusammen gemischt; alsdann purgire mit Aloen, für ein gefaundertes Pferd.

Nro. 85.

Für das Kopfweh.

Steche dem Pferd ins Maul, zwischen dem zweiten und dritten Bar, mit der Spitze deines Cornethorns oder Federmessers; laß es recht bluten und 12 Stunden stehen, dann schütte Wein oder Essig in seine Nasenlöcher, nachdem du zuvor etwas Weihrauch gegeben, laß sein Futter feucht und kühlend seyn; wenn es im Winter ist, so halte das Pferd warm.

Nro. 86.

Für weiche Hufe.

Nimm Eier und für jedes Ei einen Löffel voll Honig und für jede 2 Eier so viel gepulverten Harz, als auf der Spitze eines Sackmessers liegen bleibt; menge alles zusammen und verdicke es mit Weizenmehl; dann mache es warm und wende es Plasterweise an.

Nr. 84

For hotness in the mouth

Make a cut in the upper lip with a lancet and wash with a mixture of salt and vinegar. Then purge it with aloe for a healthy horse.

Nr. 85

For a headache

Stick the horse in the mouth between the second and third bar with the point of a corn-thorn or penknife. Let it bleed well and stand for twelve hours, then pour wine or vinegar into his nostrils. After having given him some incense, let his fodder be moist and cool. If it is in the winter, keep the horse warm.

Nr. 86

For soft hoofs

Take eggs and for every egg a spoonful of honey and for every two eggs as much pulverized rosin as can be held on the point of a pocketknife. Mix everything together and thicken it with wheat flour. Then warm it and use as a plaster.

Nro. 87.

Mit Frostbeulen behaftete Fersen.

Mische Weinhefen mit Seife zusammen wie eine Salbe, verbinde damit die wunden Stellen, und in 41 Stunden werden die Schmerzen gehoben und die Wunden geheilt seyn; die Blätter und Wurzeln von Holunder sind gut, alle jene bösen Feuchtigkeiten auszutrocknen.

Nro. 88.

Für eine vom Gebiß verletzte Zunge.

Um es zu verhindern, mache das Gebiß glatt und glänzend, und wasche es oftmals mit Lakritzensaft (liquorice), Honig und Salz; ist sie aber schon verletzt, so wasche die Zunge mit Alaunwasser oder dem Saft von schwarzen Brombeerblättern.

Nro. 89.

Auslaufende Drüsen oder morning of the chine.

Nimm Auripigmentum 2 Drachmen, ebensoviel Fassilagins pulverirt, mische es zusammen mit Terpentin zu einem Pflaster; mache kleine Kuchen daraus und trockne sie vor dem Feuer; alsdann nimm eine Kohlpfanne mit Kohlen, lege 1

Nr. 87

For chilblain affected fersen [heel]

Form a salve by mixing wine yeast together with soap. Bind up the affected part and in forty-one hours the pain is relieved and the part healed. The leaves and roots of the elder are good to dry out all that bad dampness.

Nr. 88

For a tongue injured by a bit

In order to avoid this, make the bit smooth and shiny and wash it often with licorice, honey and salt. But if the tongue is already injured, wash it with alum water or the juice from blackberry leaves.

Nr. 89

Draining glands or morning of the chine

Take two drams of *Auripigmentum* [Arsenic trisulfide, As_2S_3, from Bohemia] a like amount of powdered Tassilagins [*C. tussilaginis*] and mix them together with turpentine to form a paste. Make small cookies from this and dry them in front of the fire. Then take a brazier with coals and place one or two of the cookies on it. Cover them with a funnel and direct the smoke into the nostrils of the horse and let the smoke go into the horse's head. As soon as this is done, ride the horse until he sweats. Do this every morning before you water him until the discharge from his nose stops and the glands under his mouth have shrunk.

oder 2 Kuchen darauf, bedecke sie mit einem Trichter und lasse den Rauch durch die Nasenlöcher in des Pferdes Kopf hineingehen; sobald dieses geschehen, reite es bis es schwitzt. Dies thue alle Morgen, ehe du es tränkst, bis das Auslaufen aus der Nase aufhört und die Drüsen unter seinem Maul verkleinert sind.

Nro. 90.

Wenn das Pferd angewachsen ist, oder Auszehrung des Fleisches.

Es entspringt von übermäßigem Reisen, unregelmäßigem Futter und vielen Ueberladungen; man erkennt es durch einen allgemeinen Ekel und Magerkeit am ganzen Körper, und das Ankleben der Haut zum Körper.

Die Cur ist erstlich ein Aderlaß, und dann gib ihm 3 oder 4 Morgen zusammen jedesmal eine Quart frische Milch mit 2 Löffel voll Honig und 1 Löffelvoll grobem Theriak. Füttere es etweder mit geweichter Gerste, warmen Träbern und Salz oder mit gespaltenen Bohnen und zum Trinken Mäsches.

Nro. 91.

Milzkrankheit.

Die Milz, welches das Gefäß der Schwermuth ist, wird, wenn sie damit überladen ist, schmerzlich

D

Nr. 90

If the horse is angewachsen [emaciated] or is wasted away

The condition originates from excessive travel, irregular feeding and much overloading. The symptoms are a general nausea and poorness as well as the clinging of the skin to the body. The cure is first bleed the horse then give him every morning for three or four mornings in a row a quart of fresh milk containing two spoonfuls of honey and one spoonful of course Theriaca [a mixture of many drugs and honey]. Feed him either with softened barley, warm Träbern [fruit pulp] and salt or split beans and mash to drink.

Nr. 91

Disorder of the spleen

The spleen is the container of sadness and if it is overloaded, it becomes painfully hard and enlarged so that it is certainly visible.

The signs are much groaning, very rapid eating and a continuous looking back only on the left side.

The cure is to cook a reasonable amount of agrimony [it is an herb of the genus *Agrimonia*] in water, which the horse should then drink. Next chop the leaves up fine and mix them with butter to form a paste. Make this paste into pills and give two or three of them to the horse.

— 42 —

hart und groß, und zwar so daß es bisweilen sichtbar ist; die Zeichen sind, viel Aechzen, übereiltes Fressen und ein beständiges Hinsehen auf die linke Seite allein.

Die Cur ist also: koche eine ziemliche Quantität Odermennig (agrimony) in dem Wasser, welches das Pferd trinken soll; hacke die Blätter fein, mische sie mit Butter zu einem Teig und mache Pillen, gib dem Pferde 2 oder 3.

Nro. 92.

Eine der besten Curen für Würmer (bots).

Nimm von den weichen pflaumigen Haaren, die in den Ohren eines Pferdes wachsen und beim Scheren weggeschnitten werden, und dem kurzen Büschel, welcher oben auf seiner Stirne unter dem Vorderscheitel wächst, von jedem eine ziemliche Quantität, mische sie mit einer halben Gallon guter Hafer zusammen, und gib sie dem Pferd. — Es gibt nichts, das die Würmer mit mehr Gewißheit tödet.

Nro. 93.

Ein vortreffliches Wasser für wehe Augen, schlechtes Gesicht rc.

Nimm den Stein, genannt, Lapis calaminaris, mache ihn glühend und lösche ihn dann in

Nr. 92

The best cure for worms (bots)

Take a shears and cut some soft fine hair that grows in the ear of a horse. Take a similar amount of the short tuft that grows above on his forehead under the foremost parting of his hair. Mix these hairs together with a half-gallon of oats and give it to the horse. There is nothing that will kill the worms with greater certainty.

Nr. 93

An excellent water for sore eyes, poor eyesight, etc.

Take the stone called Lapis calminaris [impure zinc carbonate found in Alsace and Normandy], make it red hot and quench it in a half pint of white wine. Repeat this twelve times and then add one gill of house leek [Sempervivum tectorum] juice. Moisten the eye two or three times a day. It never fails.

— 43 —

einem halben Peint weißen Wein, und wiederhole es 12mal; dann setze zu 1 Tschill Hauslauchs-Saft und benetze damit das Auge 2 oder 3mal des Tags. Es fehlt nie.

Nro. 94.

Für ein Ueberbein.

Wenn die Schwiele des Ueberbeins sich nicht unterhalb der Krone des Hufs verbreitet, und ist hart und knochig; so kannst du es mit Cäustik also herausnehmen: raßire die Haare kahl ab und appliziere den Cäustik, gemacht von Kalkstein und Schmierseife, und laß ihn 24 Stunden darauf; in dieser Zeit, oder eher wenn dein Cäustik gut ist, dringt er bis zur Wurzel des Ueberbeins durch, und dasselbe kommt in 14 oder 15 Tagen rein heraus. Indeß halte Zugpflaster darauf und halte die Wunde rein von Dreck und Unrath. Wann das Ueberbein heraus ist, wende eine heilende Salbe an und wasche die Wunde mit Seifebrühe, oder Kalk- und Alaunwasser, oder Molken, alle 24 Stunden einmal frisch verbunden. Wenn wildes Fleisch sich zeigt, so brenne es weg mit Butter und Salz oder gebranntem Alaun. Wenn du sorgfältig dieses thust, so darfst du an einer Cur nicht zweifeln.

Ein Ueberbein ist im Anfange leicht kurirt, manchmal blos durch sanftes Blasenpflaster; sollte es aber hartnäckig seyn und wachsen, so appli-

Nr. 94

For bone spavin [osteoarthritic growth]

If the callous of the spavin has not spread to the under half of the crown of the hoof, you can remove it with caustic. Shave all the hair off and apply the caustic made from limestone and soft soap. Leave this on for twenty-four hours. In this time or sooner, if your caustic is good, the caustic penetrates through to the root of the spavin and the spavin comes completely out in fourteen or fifteen days. In the meantime keep the Zugpflaster [a plaster to withdraw something] on and keep the wound clean of dirt and excrement. When the spavin is out, use a healing salve and wash the wound with soapy water or lime and alum water or whey. Make a fresh dressing every twenty-four hours. If wild Fleisch [growth] appears, burn it away with butter and salt or burnt alum. If you follow this carefully, you will without a doubt effect a cure.

A Spavin in the beginning is easily cured, many times merely with a soft blatter plaster. But if the spavin is persistent and growing, apply one or two strong blatter plasters and when they are dry make an Überschlag [compress] from oatmeal, oil and vinegar. Drive the horse out to pasture. It does not fail.

zire 1 oder 2 starke Blasenpflaster und wann sie trocken sind, mache einen Ueberschlag von Hafermehl, Oel und Essig, binde denselben darauf und treibe das Pferd auf die Weide. Es fehlt nicht.

Nro. 95.

Für den Polibel.

Absud vom Snapweedöl 2 Unzen, Terpintinöl 1 Unze, mische zusammen. Es ist vortrefflich für die Fistel oder Polibel, entweder ums zu heilen wann er gebrochen ist, oder ihn zu vertreiben, oder ihn wenn er beinahe reif ist zu brechen. Es fehlt nie.

Nro. 96.

Für eine Ueberladung.

Nimm 4 Unzen von der innern Rinde der weißen Aspe, koche es in 3 Quart Wasser bis auf 2 Quart; dann nimm die Rinde heraus und löse in der Brühe 1 Unze Aloen auf, setze 1 Tschill Rum und 1 Tschill Molasses zu und gib es dem Pferd lauwarm als ein Getränk.

Nro. 97.

Böse Feuchtigkeiten zu vertreiben.

1 Pfund Feigen wohl zerstoßen mit Salz zu einer vollkommenen Salbe, vertreibt alle böse Feuch-

Nr. 95

For the polibel [poll evil]

Mix together two ounces of a concoction of snap weed [touch-me-not, *Impatiens capensis*] oil and turpentine. It is excellent for a fistula or polibel, either to heal it if it is broken or to make it disappear or to break it if it is nearly ripe.

Nr. 96

For an overloading

Take four ounces of the inner bark of the white aspen, cook it in three quarts of water until the volume has decreased to two quarts. Then take the bark out and dissolve one ounce of aloe in the broth. Add to this one gill of rum and one gill of molasses and give it lukewarm to the horse to drink.

Nr. 97

To expel bad moisture

One Pound of figs is mashed with salt to produce a salve that expels all bad moisture by opening the sweat glands and promoting the passage of the moisture.

tigkeiten, dadurch daß es die Schweißlöcher öffnet und den Durchgang befördert.

Nro. 98.

Für den Biß eines tollen Hundes.

Zuerst gib dem Pferd 2 oder 3 Löffelvoll Fünftelsaft (diapente) in Oel, Wein oder Seider; dann nimm eine lebendige Taube, öffne sie und lege sie warm auf die Wunde. Die Taube wird den Gift herausziehen, heile hernach die Wunde mit Terpentin und Schweinefett zusammen geschmolzen.

Hohlwurzblätter zerstoßen ziehen auch einigen Gift heraus; oder schabe die Wunde und thue Knoblauch und Salz hinein; es zieht das Gift heraus.—Lasse zur Ader am Halse.

Nro. 99.

Für die Auszehrung der Leber.

Nimm Schwefel und Myrrhe, ein Pfenniggewicht von jedem, stoße es zu feinem Pulver; dann nimm ein frisches Ei, stoße alles wohl zusammen und thue es in ein Peint Wein und braue es recht gut. Gib es lauwarm dem Pferde und zwar fastend. Diese Krankheit ist ansteckend.

Nr. 98

For the bite of a mad dog

First give the horse two or three spoons full of Fünftelsaft [*Diapensia lapponica*] in ale, wine or cider. Then take a living pigeon, open it and lay it warm on the wound. The pigeon pulls out the poison. After this, heal the wound with turpentine and hog fat melted together. Mashed hollow root [*Adoxa moschatellina*] leaves also extract some poisons. Or scrape the wound and apply garlic and salt. It extracts the poison. Then bleed the neck vein.

Nr. 99

For wasting of the liver

Take a penny weight each of sulfur and myrrh and pound them into a fine powder. Then take a fresh egg and pound everything together. Place this mixture in a pint of wine and brew it very well. Give this lukewarm to the fasting horse. This sickness is contagious.

— 46 —

Nro. 100.

Für Verstopfung im Körper.

Nimm Kornstroh, brühe es und mische, während es naß ist, Roggenmehl oder Kleie damit, und laß es das Pferd so heiß fressen als es kann; es wird ihm bald Luft machen.

Nro. 101.

Eine Beschreibung von unterschiedlichen der meist vorkommenden Krankheiten bei Pferden.

Wenn du die Beschaffenheit deines Pferdes Krankheit gerne ausfinden möchtest, so kehre seine Oberlippe auf eine solche Weise um, daß du sie bequem untersuchen kannst: wenn dieselbe eine weiße und knotige Erscheinung hat, so ist es durch Würmer verursacht; ist sie roth und knotig, so hat das Pferd den Engerling; ist die Lippe roth und voller Adern, so hat es die Windkolik; ist die Lippe roth ohne Adern, so hat es blos die Kolik.

Für die Curen siehe die Recepte.

Nr. 100

For constipation

Take straw and mix it with rye meal or bran while it is still wet. Have the horse eat this as hot as he can. It will give him gas.

Nr. 101

A method for differentiating the most common diseases of horses

If you want to determine the nature of your horse's sickness turn his upper lip inside out in such a way that you can easily see if it has a white and knotty appearance. If so, the illness is caused by worms. If the upper lip is red and knotty, the horse has bots. If the lip is red and full of veins, then he has wind colic. If the lip is red without veins, then he merely has colic. For the cures see the prescription.

Inhalt.

Contents

51. Stones
52. Bots
53. Blasenpflaster
54. Swelling
55. Cancer-like Swelling
56. Pinched Shoulder
57. Beginning Polibel, etc.
58. Poison, etc.
59. Dirt Malanders
60. Sweeny
61. Bots or Worms
62. Mange
63. Injured Tendon Heels
64. Brittle Hoofs
65. Mange
66. Sore Eyes
67. Blindness
68. Cancer of the Eye
69. Windgall
70. Stiff or Injured Tendon
71. Fetlock Dislocation
72. Inflammation of the Glands
73. Kidney Stones
74. Mange
75. Discharging Glands
76. Black Drink [Glands]
77. Liver Disease, etc.
78. Jaundice
79. Fetlock
80. Cramps, etc.
81. Kidneys, etc.
82. Blood Spavin, etc.
83. To Mend Broken Veins
84. Hotness in the Mouth
85. Headache
86. Soft Hoofs
87. Chilblain Affected
88. Injured Tongue
89. Draining Glands
90. Growths, etc.
91. Spleen Disorders
92. Worms [Bots]
93. Eyewash
94. Wens
95. Polibel
96. Overloading
97. Expelling Bad Moisture
98. Bite of a Mad Dog
99. Wasting
100. Constipation
101. Symptoms, etc.

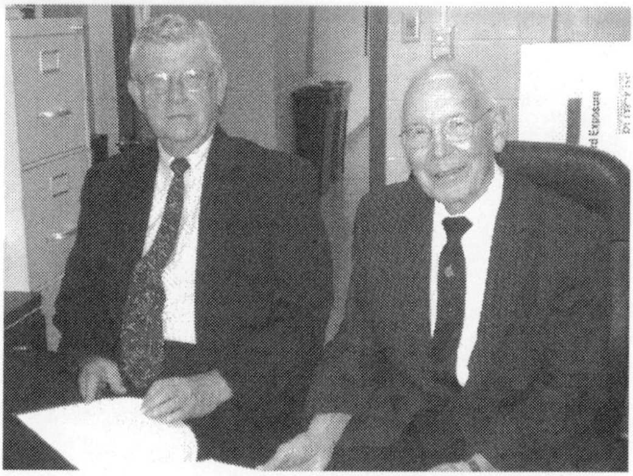

Ned D. Heindel's ancestors were Pennsylvania German farmers and cigar makers in York County, Pennsylvania. His Pennsylvania German-speaking grandmother knew many of the old country remedies, the curative chants, and the pow-wow therapies and was especially good at curing childhood hiccups. Ned took his B.S. in Chemistry at Lebanon Valley College [Annville, PA], his doctorate at University of Delaware [Newark, DE], and his postdoctoral fellowship at Princeton University [Princeton, NJ]. His research interests are in medicinal chemistry and folk-healing techniques. He is the author of the book, *Hexenkopf: History, Healing and Hexerei,* and of over 200 technical articles on drug development. He is currently the Howard S. Bunn Chair Professor of Chemistry at Lehigh University [Bethlehem, PA] where he has taught since 1966.

Robert D. Rapp was born to a Pennsylvania German family in 1930. He spent his childhood in a rural Pennsylvania German community near Reading, PA. There, at an early age, he became acquainted with the local German dialect, because his neighbors were Pennsylvania German farmers and craftsmen. After a stint in the U.S. Navy, he matriculated at Tufts University [Medford, MA] and obtained a B.S. in Chemistry in 1955. Bob worked as a chemist in industry and as a clinical chemist in the Reading Hospital before entering graduate school at Lehigh University where he was awarded a PhD in 1967. He then served as Professor of Chemistry at Albright College [Reading, PA] until his retirement in 1992. His research interests are in natural products and in medicinal chemistry. He is currently a Visiting Scientist at Lehigh University.

22851451R00079

Made in the USA
Charleston, SC
02 October 2013